# Tired Of Diets? Hate Going to A Gym? Want To Lose Weight? Let's Talk!

# Tired Of Diets? Hate Going to A Gym? Want To Lose Weight? Let's Talk!

*Kenneth R. Bibbins, Clinical Physiologist*

*&*

*Louis F. Martin, MD, F.A.C.S., F.C.C.M.*
*Bariatric Surgeon*

Writers Club Press
San Jose New York Lincoln Shanghai

Tired Of Diets? Hate Going to A Gym?
Want To Lose Weight? Let's Talk!

Writers Club Press
an imprint of iUniverse.com, Inc.

For information address:
iUniverse.com, Inc.
5220 S 16th, Ste. 200
Lincoln, NE 68512
www.iuniverse.com

ISBN: 0-595-16450-1

Printed in the United States of America

# *Contents*

# *Foreword*

It would be very suprising if anyone in this country was not aware of the alarming rise in obesity. Nowadays you can't read a newspaper, watch television, or listen to the radio without constant messages to lose weight. In 1990, there was an estimated $33 billion spent on weight loss programs. One survey found 62% of adults dieting at any given time. One would think that with the enormous amount of time and money spent on weight loss, people would be getting thinner. Yet, the U.S. Department of Health Statistics shows that Americans are getting fatter and living longer.

Let's Talk! Why are some people overweight or obese while others remain thin when consuming the same amount of food? The simple explanation given for obesity is overeating. A person becomes overweight by consistently eating more food than what is needed to maintain body weight and provide energy for their *Basal Metabolic Rate (BMR),* and general level of physical activity. Beyond this, the reasons why some people eat to the point where they become morbidly obese, a level of fatness that is life threatening, are unclear. Some obese people have been diagnosed with low functioning thyroid or slow metabolism. These conditions have a reduced basal metabolic rate. When someone does not metabolize or burn the number of calories consumed, the unused calories are stored in the body as fat. Stored body fat is used when food is unavailable as a source of energy for important bodily functions.

**In addition to these possible physiological reasons, there are a number of psychological and social reasons that people become overweight or obese. Common psychological factors that contribute to**

overeating are depression, low self-esteem, social anxiety, or poor stress management skills. Social relationships and activities also play a significant role in contributing to the development of obesity. Gathering of families, friends, and business associates often involve sharing food. Those present are encouraged to eat as a sign of being a part of the group. Eating may be a symbol of group membership. There are various reasons why one becomes overweight but no one becomes morbidly obese (when weight is more than double what it should be) without some underlying genetic factor.

Some morbidly obese people have chosen to make peace with their obesity. It is not a sign that they cannot control themselves or that they are lazy, ugly, stupid, or failures in life. Obesity is not an issue of character, intelligence, or competence. For other obese people, acceptance of their weight is not simple or sufficient. The physical, psychological, social and economic issues are significant enough for them to pursue some type of weight loss program.

The United States is in the midst of an obesity epidemic. An estimated 97 million adults in the United States are overweight or obese, conditions that substantially raise the risk of morbidity (bad health outcomes) from more than 30 comorbid conditions. Obesity related illnesses now account for an estimated 300,000 deaths per year in America, second only to tobacco related illnesses (400,000/yearly). Tobacco related illnesses however, are decreasing while the incidence of obesity is increasing, especially among children. The number of overweight Americans has increased steadily in the last decade and will continue to increase because more than 25% of today's children are overweight or obese.

As obesity specialists with years of experience in obesity research and clinical treatment programs we have had the pleasure of assisting numerous individuals fight their obesity. Obesity is a major health problem, if not the most important medical problem our society currently face. One-half of all Americans are mildly, moderately, or morbidly obese. Obese individuals are at increased risk for development of many illnesses and early death. Obese people are at greater risk for coronary thrombosis and stroke because of arteriosclerosis. They are more likely to suffer from arthritis and degenerative disease of weight bearing joints. Such people are more likely to develop diabetes, gallbladder disease, high blood pressure, respiratory insufficiency along with other medical problems. Often social and psychological stigmas are associated with obesity. Obese people may encounter unfair obstacles, such as, job discrimination, social exclusion, internalize their shame and suffer from low self-esteem.

In America, the general public has a complex relationship with the disease of obesity. Discrimination against the obese is raging, acceptable, and can best be equated to early century attitudes toward the mentally ill. Most obese individuals have attempted to lose weight multiple times but these efforts are sabotaged by various contributing factors. Their pattern of social behavior, psychological status, cultural beliefs and behaviors, each individual's physiology, their gene pool and their metabolism. This book is being written as a guide for those individuals who are tired of their sedentary lifestyle and are ready to make the lifestyle changes necessary if one is to lose weight thus bringing about wellness.

Wellness is the absence of disease resulting in optimal health. Optimal physical health should encompass choosing a healthy diet, maintaining an appropriate weight, avoiding tobacco and drug use along with other self-destructing habits, and maintaining stress effectively.

Today, many people are striving for optimal health. They are adjusting their diets, increasing their activity levels, and having physiological variables such as their blood pressure and cholesterol levels checked regularly. Afterall, the human body is designed to work best when it is physically active. It readily adapts to practically any level of activity and exertion. (The benefits of physical fitness, is the ability of the body to adapt to the demands and stresses of daily life which are physical and mental, immediate and long-term).

# *Introduction*

According to long-term studies conducted by our federal government an estimated 97 million adults in the United States are overweight or obese. Overweight is defined by the National Institute of Health (NIH), as having a Body Mass Index (BMI), equal to or greater than 30 (BMI is calculated by dividing one's weight in kilograms by the square of one's height in meters).

Obesity, is a condition that substantially raises the risk of morbidity from more than 30 conditions including cancer (breast, colorectal, prostate and endometrial) coronary heart disease, dyslipidemia, gallbladder disease, hypertension, osteoarthritis, respiratory problems, sleep apnea, strokes, and type II diabetes mellitus. Our population, already the fattest in the world, is getting fatter. As the obesity rate continues to climb, related comorbid disease rates will continue to rise as well. Costs attributable to obesity were over $90 billion in 1995 alone. Approximately $50 billion of those dollars were spent on medical care for the obese. The cost of lost productivity was $3.9 billion reflecting 39.2 million days of lost work, 239 million restricted activity days, 89.5 million bed-days, and 62.6 million physician visits in 1995. Other costs, such as human suffering, are difficult to estimate. Besides an increased incidence of associated medical diseases, the psychological effects of obesity may include lowered self-esteem, body image problems, anxiety, eating disorders and clinical depression.

Through medically supervised diet programs or fad diets obese people have sincerely tried to lose weight. Even with the help of the diet industry 95% of those who manage to shed unwanted pounds will regain them after 2 years. For some, each pound regained will take its toll in personal frustration and a sense of failure. For a morbidly obese individual who has a BMI equal to or greater than 40, the toll of those regained pounds may be especially high. Those excess pounds may lead to poor physical health, isolation, psychological distress, social prejudice, and economic discrimination.

Traditionally treatment for obesity has focused upon decreasing caloric intake and increasing physical activity. Many commercial weight loss programs have used this formula. Recognizing the psychological and interpersonal issues involved in being overweight, some medical and commercial weight loss programs include patient counselors and support groups. These diets can be depriving and are hard to stay on for very long. For some, the on-going expense of a commercial diet program can become prohibitive due to frustration, {i.e., rate of weight loss that is too slow}, response to interpersonal pressures from family and friends, or lack of money, the program is ended and the person returns to their previous eating habits and physical activity level. Usually the pounds pile back on, plus more. Dieting alienates the body from the natural process of hunger and sets you up for the real physical side efects of dieting, resulting in individuals who have learned to ignore their own survival mechanism and can lead to adaptation of an unhealthy eating regimen.

There are a number of surgical procedures designed to limit food consumption in order to facilitate weight loss. Weight loss surgery is an option for individuals whose BMI is equal to or greater than 40, or whose BMI is at least 35 with co-existing comorbidities, when less invasive methods have failed. Among these procedures are the Biliopancreatic Bypass, Gastric Bypass and the Laparoscopic Adjustable Gastric Band. Obese individuals who are contemplating surgery should understand that surgical intervention for weight loss should be a last resort. In consultation with your physician and other healthcare personnel, if it is decided that surgical intervention is the appropriate option for you, then you should view your decision for surgery as one of the initial steps in your commitment to change your lifestyle and to focus on wellness.

Body weight is dependent on the balance of caloric intake and expenditure. When energy intake and expenditure are in balance, weight remains stable. A net excess in energy, whether through caloric intake or lack of expenditure results in weight gain. When caloric intake is less than expenditure, weight loss can occur over a period of time.

Let's Talk! Like any other natural entity, the human body must obey physical law. Food is energy for the human body! This energy once consumed cannot be destroyed, only transformed. The human body's main energy storage is fat (9 grams/cal.), when your energy intake is greater than energy expenditure this unavoidably causes an increase of adipose tissue, which is always accompanied by a lesser increase of lean body mass which inevitably creates a fat weight gain. To reduce your weight there must be a change in your total energy expenditure and/or caloric intake.

Everyone has a **Basal *Metabolic Rate***, which is the energy required to maintain your vital bodily functions. Your basal metabolic rate typically accounts for approximately 55%-75% of your resting energy expenditure. Your body uses approximately 5%-15% of it's daily energy expenditure for digestion of food (diet-induced thermogenesis), which includes mastication, transport,absorption and metabolism, and the remaining 10%-40% is to be expended on your activities level (this varies greatly from individual-to-individual). Your basal metabolic rate is a tool for calculating energy needs. Calories are used as energy for bodily functions. Your resting metabolic rate (energy expenditure while resting and is usually lower than basal metabolic rate) is affected by many factors such as your age, height & weight, and gender. Energy used by increasing your activity level helps to create a caloric deficit. Increased activity levels have a positive affect on weight loss. Once you incorporate a raised level of activities into your lifestyle, you can be on your way to losing, reaching and maintaining your weight loss goal. Weight loss may be achieved and maintained with lifestyle changes such as Healthy Conscious Eating and increasing your activity levels.

# Chapter 1
# Understanding Obesity and
# It's Comorbidities

The obesity rate in most developed countries have reached epidemic proportion. Because of this alarming disease rate there is a great need to understand overweight and/or obesity. When does an overweight person become obese? Should treatment involve lifelong management incorporating diet, exercise and medication? Or, should weight loss be achieved through surgical intervention?

Let's Talk! Anyone who has a sedentary lifestyle with unhealthy eating habits is at risk for obesity. A sedentary lifestyle and obesity go hand-in-hand. Why are some people more prone to weight gain than others is a very perplexing question. Obesity has a variety of underlying causes which include differences in genetics, physiology, environment, metabolism, behaviors, caloric intake, activity level, hormone and appetite regulation in your brain.

One of the most important factors in weight gain appears to be genetic inheritance of characteristics from parents to their children. **Genetics inheritance is important for several reasons; genetics can determine the number of *fat cells* that you are born with (which may explain why some people are simply born with more of them) and create as an infant. The fat cell is ultimately the site where the changes occur in body composition and fat deposition. When your caloric intake exceeds your energy expenditure, your body will store the extra calories in fat cells that are present in *adipose tissue*.** Fat cells function as energy reservoirs, they can enlarge or decrease depending on your energy usage. When you do not balance energy output with caloric intake by adopting **healthy eating strategies and increased activity levels the fat builds up in your adipose tissue.**

These fat cells are derived from fibroblast like cells termed *adipocyte* precursors, and have the ability to multiply and enlarge. Fat cells usually multiply during two specific growth periods 1) early childhood and 2) during the hormonal changes that occur during adolescence growth period. Overeating during these time periods increases your number of fat cells (babies who are overfed become fat and often stay overweight into adulthood).

**In most cases,** after adolescence, fat cells tend to increase in size rather than number, so that adults who overeat and gain weight tend to do so because they have developed larger fat cells. Each fat cell can ballon to more than 10 times its original size, and when available cells can't hold any more fat, **the body can make new ones even in adulthood.** As your body stores more and more fat, your weight and size will increase. If this process continues, you will eventually reach the state of being overweight and/or obese (when your fat mass threatens your life and health).

Humans, have a great capacity to store food (potential chemical energy; i.e. fat/triglycerides). In historical evolutionary terms the human body's metabolism evolved so that it anticipated lean times so it conserves energy during periods of famine and stores fat for periods of abundance (harvest). This mechanism was vital to prehistoric man for survival {i.e. hunting, gathering, farming, walking, etc.} This evolutionary tendency coupled with your present day sedentary lifestyle has created excessive fat deposition in your adipose tissue. Fats that are not utilized immediately as a source of energy are stored in layers of fatty (adipose)tissue under your skin. Everyone's body contains some fat which is needed. Fat serves as cushion and protection for your vital organs and plays a role in body configuration. Also fat is stored energy in your body that can be called upon to meet your body's energy needs when other sources, particularly your blood sugar level falls. Usually, the body burns sugar (glucose) that circulates in the blood for its immediate energy needs. Your body prefers to burn glucose to satisfy its energy requirements but each period of over 6-8 hours of no food intake depletes glucose usage and encourages your body to release fat from its storage baule to meet energy requirements.

Let's Talk! Cells are the basic unit of life. All plants and animals are composed of cells. These cells are classified as either specialized or simple. A specialized cell, such as your liver, performs many complex chemical reactions. Simple cells such as your fat cells provide support and lining in your tissue. The fat cells found beneath your skin and around many of your organs are packed with triglycerides (fat). Genetic factors influence fat metabolism and regulate certain hormones and proteins (enzymes) that affect your appetite. One of these substances that play a role in obesity is Lipoprotein Lipase (LPL), an enzyme that is produced by your fat cells to help store calories as fat. If too much Lipoprotein Lipase is produced, your body will be especially efficient at storing calories. Lipoprotein Lipase is partly controlled by reproductive hormones (estrogen in women and testosterone in men), so gender-based differences in the activity of enzyme also affect development and depostition of fat. In women, fat cells in the hips, thighs, and breast secrete LPL, while in men the enzyme is produced by fat cells in the abdominal area. Fat cells in the abdominal area are believed to release their contents for quick energy usage, while fat in the thighs and buttocks are used for long term energy storage.

The complexity of weight gain mandates a multi-disciplinary approach for treatment of obesity to effect real long-term weight loss. Long-term weight loss success is based on the use of a multicare team that includes physicians and clinicians with special interest in obesity such as endocrinologists, dietitians, exercise physiologists, clinical psychologists, and behavior therapist and, when appropriate, a bariatric surgeon. The word ***"bariatric"*** is used to indicate a physician who specializes in the treatment of obesity. When planning a treatment program for weight loss you should consider your reasons for the change. Step #1, Make the decision. Step #2, Record your weight loss history and experiences with diets (this should include the time spent in each attempt and the amount of weight loss). Step #3, You also need to record your attitude toward increased activity levels, your nutritional habits (to be documented using a 2-4 day food diary history of everything you ate) and the available time you have to spend daily and weekly to implement change.

Initially, your target goal for weight loss should be a 10% weight loss over a six-month period. Your treatment strategies will need to be designed to meet the amount of help you think you will need to change your physical and nutritional habits. Your physical activity should include moderate levels of activity that you can perform continuously for 30-45 minutes for 5-7 days weekly. Your caloric intake should be based on creating a deficit of 500-1,000 calories a day under your energy needs. Your behavior can be modified via self-monitoring techniques and stress management skills to include problem solving. For morbidly obese individuals who haved reached a BMI above 40, and who have not been successful with less invasive intervention treatment options in the past, an alternative would be to examine surgical treatment options which have a high probability of letting treated individuals lose 100 pounds or more in the year after surgery. Surgical treatments are meant only for those severely obese individuals. Surgical options that are available consist of, but are not limited to are Roux-en-Y Gastric Bypass, Laparoscopic Adjustable Gastric Banding, and the Biliopancreatic Bypass. Weight loss of about 25%-60% of one's excess weight will improve metabolic and cardiovascular functioning as well as improvement in all medical conditions associated with obesity (i.e., hypertension, diabetes, arthritis, sleep apnea, leg swelling, back pain, stress incontinence, heartburn, etc.,) can be expected over the long haul as a result of losing weight due to surgery.

Regardless of the treatment option chosen, it is imperative that you increase your activity level and decrease your caloric intake. Increasing your physical activity is essential because it reduces the risk of being affected by the comorbidities of obesity such as Heart Disease, Type II Diabetes Mellitus, Stroke, and certain Cancers, all which can lead to premature disability and death. Excess weight also places stress on your bones and muscles and puts you at a higher risk for hernias, low back pain, aggravation of arthritic conditions, sleep apnea and high blood pressure.

Let's Talk! High blood pressure, or hypertension, is a contributing factor for heart disease, strokes, kidney failure and cardiovascular disease. Overweight individuals with high blood pressure are at increaserisk for enlargement of the heart, which is a major risk factor for the development of heart failure. High blood pressure is often produced when there is a need for an increased output of blood from your heart to accumulated excess tissue such as fat or resistance to normal blood flow through the arteries. The increased output or resistance is due to the altering of the physiological characteristics and function of your kidneys over time leading to a retention of sodium and water. As blood pressure rises your heart has to work harder to push the blood forward against the higher resistance. When this continues over an extended period of time your heart enlarges and the blood flow to the heart muscle becomes compromised increasing the likelihood that heart failure will develop. The major arteries which are exposed to continued levels of increased pressure thickens and this scarring hardens arteries making them less elastic. When this happens, heart attacks and strokes can occur.

Avoiding smoking and heavy drinking coupled with maintaining a healthy weight through healthy conscious eating and increased aerobic activity levels can help keep arteries elastic, which in turn, keeps blood flowing and your blood pressure low. **Being overweight can also affect your body's insulin production, which can lead to diabetes. Diabetes is a spectrum of diseases associated with insulin, the hormone that helps you maintain a healthy level of glucose. Glucose is the primary sugar your** body uses for energy, cannot be secreted in large enough quantities to satisfy the body's needs in diabetics. When your body cells do not produce enough insulin or your body's cells are prevented from receiving and using the hormone insulin {insulin resistance},the glucose level builds up in your blood—a condition referred to as *"hyperglycemia"*. Diabetes is a condition of chronic hyperglycemia that often causes very minor symptoms for years while irreversibly damaging major body organs or systems including your eyes, heart and blood vessels, brain and kidneys. Type I diabetes mellitus, which usually develops during childhood, is a condition where the insulin producing cells in the pancreas totally fail causing a loss of adequate insulin production in the body and the need for daily administration of insulin.

Type I diabetes mellitus is genetically inherited and is considered a disease of the immune system. Type II diabetes mellitus is far more common and it most often occurs in adults who are obese (Over 75% of diabetics are obese). However, Type II diabetes mellitus is now also commonly being diagnosed in very obese children, especially in Native Indian populations, certain Hispanic populations and in African American children. Type II diabetes produce some insulin but the body does not respond effectively to it and as body mass increases, insulin needs increases. Type II diabetes mellitus appears to develop in response to genetic factors (you are more at risk if you have family members with the disease) but is primarily a disease of the obese. Excess weight is believed to increase insulin resistance so diabetes can develop more easily. Type II diabetes mellitus may go on for years without major symptoms which are annoying enough to cause a physician visit. Common symptoms include frequent urination, unexplained weight loss, extreme thrist, blurred vision, fatigue and hunger. If you have a family history of type II diabetes mellitus you can often prevent the onset of the diabetes by maintaining a healthy body weight through *healthy conscious eating,* and increasing your activity levels. Healthy conscious eating (proper nutrition), and increased activity levels may have a positive effect on sleep apnea. When people become obese, the increased fat mass not only causes the outer body shape to bulge out, it also puts pressure on inner body cavities like the abdomen, brain and on the airway in the neck.

Sleep apnea, occurs when the upper throat muscles relax and the lower jaw collapse onto the airway at intervals during sleep, thereby temporarily blocking the passage of air. The sleeping individual is usually unaware of this problem but notices that he/she sleeps poorly and awakens repeatedly throughout the night. Other people in the same household will often complain about loud snoring ( a sign that the airway is collapsing causing an increased resistance to the flow of air during breathing). The symptoms of sleep apnea include morning headaches,fatigue, irritability, and waking up at night feeling you are choking. Sleep deprivation can leave you feeling tired and more prone to snacking to increase your energy level (by raising blood glucose levels), and you are less likely to increase your activity levels because you lack energy. Sleep apnea often requires medical treatment to prevent death by choking. Healthy conscious eating, and increasing your activity levels remains the essential two-fold strategy to combat the growing problems of obesity.

Extreme, restrictive diets are not the answer. Of course, if you can follow an extreme restrictive diet plan you might lose 20 or even 30 pounds initially, but this type of dieting is not a long-term strategy for maintaining weight loss. Long-term weight loss rarely occurs following severely restricting diets. The key to achieving long-term maintenance of a healthy weight is to consciously eat smaller quantities of normal healthy foods adding fruits and fibers to replace saturated fats, cholesterol and high calorie foods.

***Diets*** that produce rapid weight loss are usually not diets you can follow consistently, besides they becomes boring quickly. They do not teach practical ways for you to manage your lifestyle and weight. Most quick fix or fad diets, particularly those based on eating select foods or eating only from one or two food groups, or foods rich in protein, are not nutritionally balanced and stress the body over time.

Let's Talk! A ***calorie*** is simply the amount of heat necessary to raise the temperature of one gram of water one degree celsius to promote energy. (As you progress through the following chapters understand that the word ***calorie*** is use to describe the amount of food that your body needs to produce a unit of energy). Calories are the energy necessary for life, and your body burns a great number of calories just to maintain it's basal metabolic rate (BMR). Calories fuel your body and unused calories are stored as fat. How you lower your calorie intake/count and increase your activity level is the key! The safe way to cut calories is through healthy conscious eating, (selecting fewer foods high in fat and sugar while following a balanced meal, with selections from a wide variety of food groups).

How do you determine what your caloric needs are? Well, 3,500 calories equal one pound and by eating 3,500 more calories than your body utilizes (burn), will produce a weight gain of one pound. When you decrease your caloric storage through increased activity levels or through a caloric deficit of 3,500 calories you could lose up to one pound. This deficit is not exact, due to individual usage of calories. Think about the people you know and their eating habits. Caloric needs are estimate by having you adjust your calories either up or down until weight remains stable. Because the matter of caloric needs is personal, no two people fight the same battle. Some must cut their calories to a very low level, while others have the luxury of requiring only modest reductions. As you continue your weight loss program, you'll get a better idea of how efficient your body processes calories and what you can count on in terms of weight loss.

Losing weight is a difficult battle especially in our present day society. With the bombardment of television, magazines, and radio food advertisements; the **super-sized** take-out orders at fast food outlets; the convenience and usage of computers; the pressures of your peers to eat at social gatherings to be part of the group; **YES**, weight loss can be a battle in present day society. Yet, excess weight poses such a threat to your quality of life, health, and well-being that the battle becomes worthwhile. The battle can be won with proper support, guidance, healthy conscious eating, education and understanding, along with your commitmentand determination that results in lifestyle changes. Temporary psuedo changes will not give you the long term result you seek. If you were to eat a healthy meal six days out of the week and one day ate a very high fat, high calorie meal, your body would still try to hold onto the fat from that one meal. The worst part of this is, your body thinks it is doing you a favor by holding the fat as stored energy. A well balanced meal through healthy conscious eating provides fats, carbohydrates, proteins, vitamins, minerals, and water in the correct proportions. These nutrients must be consumed in adequate quantities to provide energy for your body.

# Chapter 2
# *Your Body's Physiological &*
# *Nutritional Needs*

Let's Talk! Definitions of body fatness or obesity, like definitions of overweight vary. Because all definitions require professional judgement when applied in individual cases, understanding the development of each definition and its use are valuable in understanding your present weight with regards to body fat versus body weight. Body fat is used to imply that some specific degree of fatness exist. Body fat is excessive to the degree that it can aggravate or manifest a comorbid medical condition such as hypertension or diabetes.

Overweight, which is defined by the National Institute of Health as having a body mass index (BMI) equal to or greater than 25 (Male or Female) implies that you are carrying more weight for your height than is healthy. In medical terms, reference to obesity and/or overweight can be defined by the presence of adverse metabolic and/or cardiovascular consequences corresponding to varying degrees of body fat. Obesity is determined by measurement of body fat not merely body weight and is also based on physical and biochemical measurements that indicate morbidity (bad health outcomes) and mortality risk. Knowing what percentage of your body weight is fat can help you determine the health risk associated with your weight. Your health risk history is based on three physical measurements; weight for height, body fat, and regional body fat distribution. Overweight refers to an excess amount of total weight including all tissues. For men the definiton refers to a weight that is 20% above "Ideal Body Weight" (IBW), and for women, 25% above "Ideal Body Weight" (IBW). Ideal body weight has been determined by the insurance industry as the weight for each height of individual who lives the longest.

Obesity refers specifically to an excess of body fat and can be measured in several ways. For example,in most instances men and women **with a BMI equal to or greater than 25 are considered *overweight*. If your body mass is equal to or greater than 30, then you are considered *obese*. The term obesity, in contrast to overweight, is defined as enough excess body fat to begin adversely affecting your health.**

Ideally, it would be best to measure the size and number of fat cells to provide a good profile of your obesity. Watching fat cells decrease in size would be a strong motivating tool. However, outside of the research laboratory, the procedure for obtaining fat cells is **impractical and expensive making other measurements of body fat which are more safe and pain free more practical. Practical methods currently used are BMI calculation, skin fold calibers and bioelectrial impedance apparatus to measure your fat mass. Excess fat accumulation is associated with an increase in the cell size of the fat cells, referred to as *hypertrophic obesity*. The other type of obesity that exist is referred to as *hypercellular obesity*, where the number of fat cells** also increases but this is rare in adults. Fat cell distribution refers to patterns of body fat located in different regions of the body, such as central and truncal locations.

Most research evaluating how the distribution of fat cells affect health has shown central obesity is more hazardous to your health than truncal obesity which appears to be more benign. Fat cell turnover maybe related to the health consequences for those with central (abdominal) obesity "apple-shaped" (men). Central fat is of two kinds; subcutaneous, and visceral. The visceral fat in the central region seems to have much more rapid turnover than the sluggish subcutaneous fat in the truncal region. Also visceral fat seems to increase with age in both genders in lean as well as obese individuals. Those with truncal or peripheral fat are called "pear-shaped" (women). Women usually have pear shaped obesity adding stores of fat to their hips, buttocks and thighs, especially during pregnancies.

Healthy body composition involves a high proportion of lean body tissue and acceptable levels of body fat, adjusted for age and sex. Since gaining weight is partly genetic and leads to chronic medical problems it is important to continously work at preventing it. When attempting to lose weight you will see your weight flucuate; it drops, then stabilizes, before dropping more. Alternatively, you may have a relapse when old habits prevail and you regain the weight you lost.

Over time, immediate, short-term adjustments translate into long-term changes and improvements. There is a graded inverse relationship between physical activity and mortality (Research demonstrates that healthier people live longer). The benefits of maintaining a healthy weight are both physical and mental, immediate and long term. Maintaining a healthy body weight can allow you to do everyday tasks, such as walking, climbing stairs and lifting with less exertion, providing you with the reserve strength needed for emergencies. Increased activitity levels helps reduce body fat and helps control body weight. This all helps the body in preventing disease, thus bringing about wellness. Appropriate goals to focus on more than just weight loss or body fat loss, are approaches that can produce improved health benefits independently of weight loss. Health is improved by increasing physical activity, by making qualitative changes in food consumption, and by eliminating destructive habits especially cigarette smoking. Measuring success in weight loss is not measuring the amount of weight loss during a relatively short period of time. Long term amelioration of medical problems, better health coupled with an improved quality of life, with or without extreme weight loss are the most important measures of success.

When increasing your activity levels and implementing a plan to promote healthy conscious eating, you need to match your eating and activity plans with your physical and financial limitations, level of motivation, pre-existing medical condition, utilizing your past history of weight loss attempts to help you make more appropriate plans and realistic goals. A great deal of time must be spent initially on deciding the best course of action for you. Realize physical activity or adhering to a increased activity training program may not make all people lean. Lifestyle behavioral change must occur to obtain long-term weight loss. Several ways to achieve behavioral change resulting in weight loss are to increase activity levels, practice good nutritional eating and learn how to manage stress effectively.

In today's world, some people often eat as a response to peer pressure in social settings. Others eat for comfort or as a response to other emotions such as anger, loneliness, frustration, rejection, etc. These settings are unavoidable in most instances and should not be shied away from. It is more important to have mechanisms in place to make the proper adjustments to foods in your daily life. Once you begin to utilize healthy conscious eating principles in relation to caloric intake and caloric expenditure you can have better control of your weight loss/maintenance plan. Obesity prevention is within everyone's grasp. It begins with the promotion of healthy eating habits and increasing activity levels. Interventions can be as simple as watching less television, walking more often and decreasing your caloric intake.

Let's Talk! Caloric intake is simply the amount of food you consume, usually calculated daily. Although common sense suggests that overeating is involved in any weight gain, yet, research has not shown a direct correlation with caloric intake and obesity. In fact, there is no sound evidence demonstrating that obese people eat more than people who are not obese. Simply stated, regardless of how many calories you previously consumed daily, to lose weight you must decrease your caloric intake according to your weight loss goals and activity levels. Caloric intake must equal your caloric expenditure for you to maintain stable weight. When your caloric intake is less than your expenditure you will lose weight. When your caloric intake is more than your caloric expenditure, you will gain weight. Food intake should serve three major purposes; 1) It is used to regulate body processes 2) The components of food may be used to build, repair or maintain body tissue and, 3) Food is to be used as energy.

Let's Talk! All energy comes directly from the sun. Simple elements from the earth and surrounding air such as carbon dioxide, water, minerals and salts provide energy for plants to grow and reproduce. These elements are converted into complex food materials, which are subsequently broken down for energy. Your body cannot convert these simple elements into energy so you have to derive this nourishment directly from either plants, or the animals that have eaten the plant

**Foods eaten are considered "energy-in." Activity levels are considered "energy-out." Energy-in takes the form of three basic nutrients; carbohydrates, fats, and protein. These three nutrients supply energy for your body. Your body breaks these nutrients down and energy is released. Simple carbohydrates as well as complex carbohydrates supply four calories of energy per gram and are composed of carbon and water. Simple carbohydrates provide much of the sweetness in foods and can be a source of readily available energy (fresh fruit). Your liver breaks down complex carbohydrates such as dietary fibers and starches before they can be used by your body as energy. Atoms of carbon, hydrogen, and oxygen combine to form a sugar molecule (A carbohydrate), referred to as glucose.**

**During digestion, the body breaks down complex carbohydrates (two-sugar molecules) into simple carbohydrates (one-sugar molecules). Carbohydrates are then absorbed by your small intestine and broken down by your liver into glucose,(also called dextrose or blood sugar). Glucose (which is a natural sugar in food) is then absorbed into your blood stream and used as energy by your body; stored in your muscles and liver as glycogen; or converted to lipids (fat) for energy storage. Carbohydrates serve important functions in your body with relation to metabolism and** activity levels and is an important factor in determining how much fat will be burned and how much will be retained. In fact, the primary function of carbohydrates is to serve as fuel for your body which reduces your body's need to use fat as a fuel.

Carbohydrates are stored in limited quantity in your liver and muscles and also serves as a primary and major source of energy in order to spare the breakdown of your body's protein. Carbohydrate intake usually has a direct impact on weight gain or loss. Basically once the capacity of the cell for glycogen storage is reached, excess sugars are converted to and stored as fat. Carbohydrates consumed in excess of your activity levels are stored as fat. Conversion of carbohydrates to fat allows you to build up a fat reserve. It has been believed that occassional excess carbohydrate consumption can readily be converted into stored body fat. It has now been established that the occassional consumption of unsually high amounts of carbohydrates can be handled by temporary expansion of glycogen stores. To induce fat gain your body's total glycogen stores must first be enhanced accordingly. To produce rates of fat formation exceeding the rate at which fat is burned your total glycogen stores must first be raised substantially. This requires deliberate and sustained over consumption of large amounts of carbohydrates. A few days of fat deposition or mobilization hardly affects the size of your fat storage, which are usually over 10 kg (9000 kcal) in most adults. It is not uncommon to accumulate 20kg (44 pounds) of stored fat when you become overweight. Obese people accumulate an energy reserve 100 to 200 times greater than all the body's glycogen stores.

**Fat is stored in special cells, which become enlarged and are bigger than most of the body's other cells. Fat cells can expand or shrink considerably, but once formed, only their size, not their number can be reduced by fasting and/or dieting. Oils and fats in plants and animals are *lipids* known as triglycerides. Triglycerides are stored in depots known as adipose or fat tissue, where they make up approximately nine *kilocalories* per tablespoon. Energy is stored in adipose tissue with about 8 kilocalories in each gram of tissue which makes it possible for individuals to carry a substantial energy reserve. In lean adults, fat reserves which typically amount to about 5 kilograms (11 pounds),**

which is an energy reserve of forty-five thousand kilocalories, enough to survive about one month of near-total food deprivation.

When your caloric intake exceeds your energy expenditure your body will store the extra calories in your fat cells. When you do not balance your energy output with your caloric intake, a weight gain will occur. It is vital to eat healthy and to increase your activity levels for increased metabolic response. Daily carbohydrate consumption (thermic effect 10%), should be enough to maintain your body's store of glycogen (total glycogen stored in your body is only 100 GM or 400 kilocalories. This amount of glycogen will last less than 24 hours of fasting). This is where a lot of people usually get into problems. Americans typically consume 40% to 50% of their total calories as carbohydrates. This is generally in the form of fruits, grains, and vegetables.

This brings us to one of many explanantions why diets fail. Glucose is essential for the proper functioning of your **Central Nervous System** (CNS). In normal situations and in short-term starvation, your brain uses blood glucose almost exclusively as its fuel and essentially has no stored supply of glucose. Your brain depends almost exclusively on glucose to obtain its energy, requiring about 5 grams of glucose per hour, or 120 grams per day in adults. During fasting or starvation or with just low carbohydrate intake, your body's metabolism undergoes an adaptation after 8-10 days so that your brain uses a relatively large amount of fat in the form of acetoacetate for its fuel. By not giving your body enough carbohydrates at rest or even during increased activity levels you are unable to sustain a constant blood glucose level and that level eventually falls below normal (70-100 mg/dl).

Your glucose level must be sufficient enough in your blood to allow for diffusion into your cells to support metabolism. If your blood glucose level falls below normal your central nervous system does not have enough fuel to function. The symptoms of this condition (hypoglycemia) consist of weakness, hunger and dizziness. Sustained and profound low blood sugar levels can cause loss of consciousness and irreversible brain damage.

Because of the important role of glucose in nerve tissue metabolism, blood sugar is usually regulated within narrow limits and should be monitored and closely watched during periods of fasting or increased activity levels. As you increase your activity levels you should consume about 60% of your daily calories (400-600 grams) as carbohydrates, predominately in the unrefined complex form to prevent carbohydrate deficiency. A carbohydrate deficient diet rapidly depletes muscle and liver glycogen and can profoundly affect both aerobic and anaerobic activites.

There are three kinds of carbohydrates; monosaccharides (sugars such as glucose and fructose); oligosaccharides (disaccharides such as sucrose, lactose, and maltose) and polysaccharides that contain three or more simple sugars to form starch, fiber, and glycogen. When your diet is insufficient in carbohydrates to satisfy the needs of the brain and red blood cells, your body will attempt to make its own from protein causing a loss of *lean muscle mass.* Your metabolic rate is directly related to your lean body mass, the higher your lean body mass the higher your metabolic rate. Adequate carbohydrate intake prevents your body from using protein, the body's basic building blocks as fuel/energy.

Proteins are important, the *thermic effect* of digesting and metabolizing protein is approximately 25% of its energy content (Remember food is energy and it requires energy usage to chew and digest). The word *protein* is derived from the greek word meaning "prime importance." Protein is a muscle builder and metabolizes three times quicker than fat does and serves a vital role in skeletal structure, issue maintenance repair and growth. So when possible you should avoid losing protein (lean muscle mass). Since glycogen reserves can become **reduced or even depleted in starvation periods or in diets with reduced carbohydrate intake, it is advisable to increase your daily protein intake when dieting or when you decrease your carbohydrate intake. Protein is an important component of muscle, bone, and blood enzymes and some hormones.**

**Protein is a vital nutrient that your body needs to assist with metabolism and is similar to carbohydrates and fat by their chemical**

make-up with the addition of nitrogen. Proteins provide 4 calories of energy per gram and are composed of amino acids. The three major sources of body proteins are blood plasma, visceral tissue and muscle. Your body doesn't have a reservoir of protein because all proteins are either part of tissue structure or exist as an important aspect of metabolism.

Try to avoid losing large amounts of protein during your weight loss efforts. Protein makes up between 12%-15% of your body's mass. Usually, the brain cell contains about 10% protein, red blood cells and muscle cells contain as much as 20%. The protein content of skeletal muscle, which represents about 65% of the body's total protein, increases with weight training. Your body needs protein which is essential for growth and tissue repair and are referred to as amino acids. There are thousands of combinations of *amino acids,* but for our purpose we will concentrate on *essential amino acids,* and *non-essential amino acids.*

Let's Talk! There are eight amino acids that cannot be synthesized by the adult body and must be derived from food. These amino acids can be found in plants and animals. Proteins are considered low quality or incomplete if they do not provide all the essential amino acids, which includes products such as beans, nuts, and peas. The golden rule to remember is, if protein comes from an animal it is considered "high quality" or "complete," if it comes from a plant it is considered "low quality" or "incomplete." Usually about 10 to 15 percent of total calories should come from protein daily. Excess consumption beyond this percentage is not harmful to a degree, but remember it will be synthesized into fat for energy storage or usage. Remember to eat slowly allowing at least 20-30 minutes to complete a meal. Food that contain the proper nitrogen balance (egg, milk, meat, fish and poultry) are essential for tissue growth and repair and should be referred to as complete proteins. Incomplete proteins lack one or more of the essential amino acids. Diets containing incomplete protein usually results in protein malnutrition. This can happen even though your diet is adequate in caloric intake. Good meal planning for adequate protein intake means planning in terms of the whole meal. Think of various foods in combination as opposed to in terms of individual selections. Remember intake protein to spare lean muscle mass.

When pursuing a weight loss plan one should participate in strength training. Strength training improves body composition by increasing lean muscle mass. Increased lean muscle mass through strength training helps with reducing fat weight due to the increased metabolism. Your metabolic rate is proportional to your lean body mass. The more lean muscle mass you have, the higher your metabolic rate. A healthy body composition means that the body has a high proportion of lean muscle mass and a relatively small porportion of fat. Remember your body does need some fat. Body fat is important for many reasons. It protects your vital organs from shock, it provides insulation and warmth, is involved in the production of hormones, and fat does provide 9 calories of energy per gram and is considered the most concentrated source of energy when utilized, but too much body fat results in obesity. A good question to pose to yourself when preparing or eating a meal would be, "Do I really need as much energy as I'm about to consume?"

Weight management interventions are predicated on behavioral changes that constitute a healthy lifestyle, and potentially influence your weight status. Muscle weighs more than fat, but takes up less space. The combination of increased activity; strength training, and proper nutrition can result in a reduction of body fat not necessarily body weight. In essence a weight loss program can result in lost inches and decrease body fat percentage and not necessarily a large amount of body weight lost body weight. Reducing body fat by reducing inches is a good way to measure your weight loss efforts.

Increased activity levels need not be strenuous to be beneficial. Build up your endurance time gradually, starting out with as much time allowed by your current fitness level. Your goal is to work your way up, eventually, from an easy to a moderate-to-vigourous level that increases your breathing and heart rate. Moderate amounts of daily physical activity can be helpful for people of all ages. Increases in your activity level can be obtained with activities such as brisk walking, jogging or routine house chores.

Activities like walking and jogging are cardiorespiratory activities that require lots of oxygen as your muscles burn calories. Aerobic activities, such as walking and/or jogging, when consistently done, can lead to a more efficient cardiorespiratory system. It increasing the efficiency of your heart and strengthen your skeletal system. If you have been sedentary for quite some time it is advisable that you begin your weight loss program by walking, which is less strenuous on your weight bearing joints than jogging. Once you are able to walk relatively comfortable at a sustained pace for approximately 30 minutes, you should next begin to monitor your target heart rate.

The *Target Heart Rate (THR)*, as a calculated range and level of exertion that you should exercise at to achieve maximal results.

To Calculate Your Exercise Target Heart Rate (THR), and Resting Heart Rate (RHR), count your pulse at the carotid artery on your neck or on the inside of your wrist using the first two fingers on one hand. Count your pulse for 15 seconds and multiply that number by 4. This is your resting heart rate. To calculate your exercise Target Heart Rate & Target Heart Rate Exercise Percentage use the equation below: **Example:** 24 year old **female walking 1.0 mile a sustained pace at 60% THR.**

220-24=196 (maximal beats per minute=Target heart rate)

196 x 50%=98 beats per minute    (Sedentary to Active)

196 x 60%=117.6 beats per minute(Able to sustain 30 minutes)

196 x 70%=137.2 beats per minute        (Begin monitoring THR)

196 x 80%=156.8 beats per minute        (Moderate work-out)

196 x 85%=166.6 beats per minute(Vigorous sustained work-out)

The Target heart rate is a method of calculating the intensity of your efforts. It is a way for you to measure your intensity level with relation to progressive overload so that you stress your body enough so that change

occurs over time. *Caution: If you have a long standing medical condition (i.e., irregular heart beat, congestive heart failure) or take medications that affect your heart rate*
**(DO NOT USE THE TARGET HEART RATE METHOD).**

# Chapter 3
# The Role of Food in Your Body

Let's Talk! Some of your struggles may be genetics, and some of your struggles maybe culture, habit, or a combination of all three. There are distinct patterns of overeating associated with obesity. For instance, the degree of stress to which you are subjected to at the time the eating occurs, the environment and present of others. We understand the establishment of a particular eating pattern is probably multi-factorial in nature. One way that may lead to a healthier lifestyle and eating behavioral change is to increase your activity levels and decrease your caloric intake through Healthy Conscious Eating, this will allow you to eat a larger variety of foods in an effort to combat nutritional boredom.

Another approach would be to continue your present activity levels and adhere to a stricter food base. Changing your current eating habits to a Healthy Conscious Eating regimen where you consume more whole foods may allow you to eat more, while decreasing your caloric intake. This is attributable to a two-thirds reduction in fat intake. It also doubles your fiber intake. Eating whole foods eliminates about 340 calories a day from your diet, which can cause a decrease of 3 pounds of fat weight a month alone.

Healthy conscious eating involves more than food selection, counting calories, or eating low fat foods. It also means eating the right portion sizes and at the right times. Breakfast should be your first meal of the day and should be consumed within 30 minutes after awakening. Breakfast refuels your body by restoring your glucose level. Remember, glucose is the primary fuel source that your brain needs for functioning. Eating breakfast can improve your energy level and concentration.

Breakfast offers a nutritional advantage as well. Individuals who eat breakfast foods, such as cereal, get more carbohydrates, fiber and other nutrients and less fat and cholesterol in their diets than people who consume other types of breakfast foods or who completely skip breakfast altogether. Eating breakfast benefits your weight loss efforts by assisting you in preventing *hunger backlash*. If you continuously skip breakfast and eat later in the day, usually you have the tendency to overeat. Some individuals believe that by skipping breakfast they are saving themselves calories over the course of the day. This is absolutely not true; actually skipping breakfast may slow down your metabolism. Skipping breakfast causes your body to become caloric efficient and affects the rate your body burns calories, which could potentially cause a weight gain because your body will hold onto food if it is not replenished.

It is advisable to have a snack after breakfast followed by a balanced lunch. Lunch like any other meal should contain a balance of simple carbohydrates for immediate energy and a moderate amount of protein with a minimal amount of fat. Simple and complex carbohydrates are a good mix for your lunch time meals. If you are like most individuals you are busiest during the middle of the day, so you would definitely need to replenish the expended calories from your body. You do not want to skip lunch or consume a lunch to high in fat and not enough energy that causes you to feel fatigued afterwards.

Most of you can recall that usually after eating you tend to feel drowsy and are ready for immediate rest or sleep. This happens because when you consume a large amount of calories during any meal more blood is drawn toward your intestines to assist with the transport of the nutrients throughout your body. This causes a reduced blood flow to your brain, this coupled with other factors related to digestion, may make you drowsy. Eating five to seven times daily in smaller caloric amounts is a better way to replenish your energy needs. Eating smaller meals throughout the day may also fit better into your busy day or lunch period. Eating several small meals throughout the day should replenish your energy needs and stave off hunger until dinner. Dinner should also consist of a balanced meal that contains carbohydrates, proteins and low fats. This meal should be low in calories. Remember "food–in" is considered energy, ask yourself, *"Do I really need as much energy for my night time activities and vital bodily functions as the evening winds down?"* Most of you would answer, "NO!" Eating a modest breakfast, a little mid-morning snack, a modest lunch, a little mid-afternoon snack can assist you with controlling your hunger at dinner time; and help you to avoid late night snacking and/or bingeing.

If you are morbidly obese late night snacking and/or bingeing should definitely be avoided. Overweight and obese individuals are at increased risk for heartburn and/or Gastroesophageal Reflux Disease (GERD). Pressure on your abdomen caused by excess weight can contribute to the acid that is in your stomach to back up into your esophagus, commonly called your food pipe. When it escapes into your esophagus, through a weak or overloaded valve at the top of your stomach the result is heartburn or acid reflux. This back-up causes a powerful burning sensation felt at the back of your throat and chest when you belch. This is caused by the powerful stomach acid that has escaped. Lying flat can produce intense acid reflux after meals. Often this occurs at night, especially after a late meal, and if you are asleep when this occurs, the regurgitated acid may be inhaled, causing a searing of the airway, violent coughing and gasping. This condition is dangerous, because of the possibility of pneumonia or lung injury. If you suffer from this, you should avoid late night eating, lifting, bending over, or napping after a meal. Chronic heartburn sufferers should take a walk or remain upright after meals. Chronic heartburn or acid reflux may be managed with lifestyle and dietary changes. If chronic conditions persist you should consult your physician.

How much and what you eat is usually determined by the time and the way you eat. Everyone has a comfortable time and a preferred manner in the way they eat. Some people hurriedly eat while never really tasting or enjoying their food, while others eat considerably slower allowing for the ***satiety*** signal to arrive at the brain (usually 20-30 minutes). Some people pick at their food, others gobble everything up in chunks; and then there are still others who have no problem leaving food on their plates—they simply stop eating when they are full. Still others feel obliged to consume everything that is in front of them. Other factors to consider are the foods that are served due to culture preferences, how long you sit at the dining table and how much time you allow yourself to eat.

If you are a person who eats on the run, you often find yourself sneaking in meals at fast food places. In the mornings, if you are hurrying, you probably routinely pull into a fast food drive-through place for a quick-menu breakfast that is usually high in fat content. For lunch, it may be the same fast pace scenario, where you constantly find yourself at a fast food drive-through restaurant ordering a "super-sized" order of whatever appeals to your appetite/hunger at that time. For dinner, it is usually the same hurried pattern where the family dinner consist of high-calorie, high-fat pre-packed foods, or even worse, the family decides to order from a delivery place that specializes in quickly prepared, high fat content foods.

Let's Talk! Eating is one of the oldest habits you have and certain habits can create problems for you when compared to your activity level and present lifestyle. If you eat too fast you fool your body's satiety system. How does your body decide when you are full? Certain hormones secreted by the stomach and intestine are known to contribute to satiety, which is the feeling of satisfaction and fullness. When you eat, the food is digested, your stomach and intestines release hormones into the blood stream, which acts as messengers to your brain. When the hormones reach the hunger center of your brain, they deliver the message that sufficient food has been consumed. Various parts of the brain, including a small portion at the base of the brain called the hypothalamus play a large role in this determination. Your eating patterns are regulated by feeding and satiety centers located in your hypothalamus and pituitary glands. They respond to signals indicating when your fat cells are full. It is believed (a study conducted in mice; not yet proven to be fact in humans), the enzyme leptin is released by your fat cells. The amount of leptin produced by your fat cells appears to indicate to your hypothalamus when your fat cells are full or not. The leptin level rises as more fat is stored in your fat cells. The rising levels appear to signal your hypothalamus to suppress your appetite and when leptin levels are lowered it signals your hypothalamus to stimualte your appetite. Your levels of body fat storage can be reduced over time with consistent healthy conscious eating and increased activity levels.

Healthy Conscious Eating, active living and behavioral change can be vital components of a weight loss program. Decide what is best for you, remember what may be good behavioral changes for one may ultimately be bad behavioral changes for someone else. Behavior is a learned response to specific experiences, education, preparation and perceptions. Positive consequences usually reinforce the behavior. The first step in behavioral change in regards to getting control of your eating habits would be to begin and keep an accurate record (food diary), of the foods that you are currently eating and the times that you are eating them. You are probably saying to yourself as many people do, "I am already aware of what I am eating; why should I have to record it?"

Well, because as the saying goes, "Seeing is believing!" When you can pinpoint the times and the amount of calories you are consuming you can better develop a plan to make the necessary adjustments to meet your energy needs. By utilizing the recorded food diary you can identify your stimuli to eating. Once they have been identified, you can begin working on minimizing the effects the cues have on your food consumption. Paying close attention to your food diary entries with relation to the times that you are eating, the locations where you are eating, your emotional state when you eat, and the degree to which you experience hunger prior to eating can be helpful in exploring new ways to reduce the number of external cues that trigger your hunger and to implement new non-food responses to those cues.

The initial steps in replacing old behavioral habits with new behavioral habits are motivation and direction. You must be mentally prepared to resist the temptations that you will eventually encounter. To establish motivation that is worthy of the sacrifice and to keep you balanced and focused in the battle of weight management; ask yourself this question, "What is it that I want to do that I am unable to do, because of my health and weight?"

Goals are very important in weight loss/maintenance efforts. Some individuals fall prey to the belief that once they lose the desired weight, keeping it off will be easy. Set specific short-term and long-term goals (see Appendix E). If you have no plan or goals you cannot measure the progress in your change process. Change your behavior from a reactive position to a pro-active position, whereas your behavior is directed at a certain result. Change is not an event but a process of stages culminating in a desired result. The 1st stage that you encounter when effecting change is the thinking/contemplating stage, this is when you are considering making a behavioral change because you desire a different or a specific result, yet, you have not taken any actual steps toward realizing this change. You could spend quite a bit of time in this stage and most will. The 2nd stage usually is commitment, this is when you have made the decision to effect a change and have defined the exact steps and formulated a plan (whether alone or with help) needed to make the desired change. The last stage is action, this is when you actually put your plan into action and have taken concrete steps to reaching your desired result. You need a detailed plan and a systematic approach to weight loss. Decreasing calories through Healthy Conscious Eating, and increasing your activity levels are the ultimate steps in a weight loss/maintenance plan. Referring to your resting metabolic rate, the calories in your weight loss diet will be different from the calories in your weight maintenance diet. It is very difficult to limit calories for an extended period of time, especially for people who have the habit of continuously overeating. (Managing weight loss can be as challenging as you allow it to be). It is very important to understand that permanent weight loss requires Healthy Conscious Eating, increased activity levels and lifestyle changes; also you should be forewarned that decreasing caloric intake can be difficult.

If you do not develop new or additional coping skills for handling stress effectively and a better understanding of your body's nutritional needs and health maintenance; you can fall prey to the weight cycling, where the weight is an off-again, on-again, off-again, on-again cycle. Another important reason for staying with or committing to an active lifestyle change for continued weight loss and behavior modification,is psychological motivation. People who reach their goal weight, only to have the pounds creep back on find that experience somewhat depressing. The effort and commitment it took to lose the unwanted pounds and to see the weight reappear can be scary for most. Perhaps the thought of having to start all over again is traumatic, because each time you lose fat weight and regain that weight it becomes harder and harder to lose the fat weight again due to the disproportional fat/lean ratio of the regain.

Food consumption is determined by the habitual pattern of meals, complimented, when necessary, by physiological regulatory mechanisms, which ensures that glycogen reserves are sufficient to avoid hypoglycemia. (One of the many health reasons for keeping excess weight off). Scientific evidence strongly suggests that overweight individuals who lose relatively small amounts of their excess weight sometimes find that an accompanying comorbid disease lessens or may even disappear.

New and old methods and regimens for weight loss are constantly promoted. Some regimens are based on sound advice and principles and others on unsupported claims. Energy expenditure is correlated with body size. Once weight has been lost, weight maintenance energy (calories) will need to be reduced. A low fat diet generally allows a steady state of body weight maintenance to become established at a lower degree of adiposity. A sharp reduction in fat intake can therefore be expected to lead to a reduction of adipose tissue mass in individuals previously consuming substantial amounts of fat. To be effective as a measure for weight loss/maintenance, a reduction in fat intake must be substantial and complimented by efforts to limit carbohydrate intake. (Avoidance of food with substantial fat content has the disadvantage of restricting food choices).

Many diets that promote weight loss consist of intaking 1,000—1,500 calories daily without stressing major shifts in the relative proportions of carbohydrate, fats, and proteins. This is why healthy conscious eating is a better approach when attempting weight loss as opposed to dieting. Shifts in energy intake are imperative during weight loss. Balanced selection and control of portion sizes, while developing knowledge about foods and control of eating behavior is essential for long-term success in weight loss. A good way to reduce the body's fat content is to use it as fuel by increasing your activity levels.

Fat metabolism is limited to the gap between energy expenditure and carbohydrate and protein intake, extensive restriction of carbohydrate intake is essential to induce rapid fat loss. Near avoidance of carbohydrates forces the body to meet most of its energy needs by burning fat. Depending on body size and activity level this can induce metabolism of 150 to 250 grams of fat per day. Total carbohydrate starvation creates the greatest energy deficit and a good initial weight loss, due to decrease in extra-cellular volume during the first days of carbohydrate deprivation, but beware there is a great disadvantage to total starvation and total liquid diets. These types of diets cause a major loss of body protein, electrolytes and, potassium. Total starvation diets also has unpleasant side effects such as fatigue, hair loss from lack of protein intake, and possible gallstone formation due to the fat not being broken down properly and diposed of. Also, most of your initial weight loss will be in fluids and minerals. Some fat is lost along with muscle (protein), (Another reason why adopting a Healthy Conscious Eating behavior is optimal opposed to adhering to a restrictive diet program). Your muscle loss can be up to 30% of the total weight loss causing a decrease in your metabolism. Such losses can be minimized by consuming protein in the form of protein shakes or protein meal replacement bars. Prolonged starvation can be tolerated for several days, as the liver produce ketone bodies to replace glucose as fuel for your brain. (Ketone is a substance formed by your body during the breakdown of fats and fatty acids into carbon dioxide and water; excessive amounts of ketones are formed when fat is used instead of glucose for energy). Ketone bodies can cause nausea, bad breath and lightheadedness.

While weight reduction depends on defeating the natural tendency to regulate food intake, in weight maintenance you should be able to rely to some extent on spontaneous control of food consumption, or at least minimize the struggle against increased intake. It is therefore important to recognize that the logic for nutrient selection during weight maintenance and weight reduction are different. To avoid weight gain, it is necessary and sufficient for an individual to burn as much fat as one eats. This is extremely hard when consumption of diets with substantial amounts of fats is coupled with a sedentary lifestyle. If you fail to limit your fat intake or fail to maintain adequate low glycogen stores to facilitate fat metabolism your adipose tissue mass will expand. High glucose/insulin prevents your fat cells from releasing fatty acids into your blood stream where they can be picked up by other tissues and metabolized. Remember, metabolism is the method by which your body processes food into energy and then uses that energy for expenditure and your vital bodily functions. The dangers from obesity are not from simply being overweight; they arise from the presence of too much fat. Healthy Conscious Eating and strength training activities to increase muscle mass, are the critical components for any weight control program. Increased activity levels are essential in keeping your body fat down. As long as your eating habits and activity levels are unchanged, your body weight and body configuration will remain unchanged.

# Chapter 4
# Nutrition for Energy During Weight Loss

Let's Talk! It's true some people become overweight and/or obese while others remain thin when consuming relatively the same number of calories. This can be attributed to a variety of factors such as physiological, psychological, environment and genetics which play significant roles in determining weight distribution and accumulation. Understanding your body and weight gain is a multi-factorial task. The human body hasn't undergone any significant changes within the last 100,000 years or so. Replenshing energy for the body was then, and is now required every 2 to 2 ½ awaken hours.

Food will always be a part of society and will always have its place at social settings, celebratory events, as well as periods of mourning in different cultures. Some first dates and business meetings are places where lunch or dinner are the social settings. Because of societal norms, it is imperative that you utilize education with regards to caloric intake and expenditure. You should not allow the ideas of others to determine how you feel about yourself. It is that sort of public empowerment that can lead to stress, depression and eating disorders.

Faddish ideas, television, and clever marketing ploys cause some people to feel that no matter how much weight is lost it is never enough. Many people who are prone to obesity may not be overeaters but may be undereducated regarding information needed to make better choices. Food is nothing more than energy, yet food is used in a variety of other ways that encourages you to overeat at social settings to "fit-in." Some individuals use food for comfort when they are frustrated, tired, bored or depressed, while others find solace in the pleasant taste of food or "high calorie" drinks at the end of a hard day. Because of the important role of food in your body, you need to better understand it's purpose and how to best utilize food in healthier ways. Food is here to stay and should not be avoided. When embarking on a healthier lifestyle, it can be approached in different ways. With proper information and other coping skills dieters can begin to shift their strategies from avoidance of certain foods to consciously eating all foods that they enjoy in moderation, at appropriate times, geared toward specific results. Healthy Conscious Eating coupled with better/additional understanding of food consumption can assist you with your individual reliance, obsession and consumption of food. A good dietary approach for successful healthy weight should encompass the following:

1) Food selection should meet all nutritional needs for energy.
2) Food selection should eliminate nutritional boredom.
3) Food selection is conducive to improvement of overall health.
4) Food selection meets individual taste and habits.
5) Food should be readily obtainable and socially acceptable.
6) Food should favor a positive changed eating pattern.
7) Food selection should encompass Healthy Conscious Eating.

You derive pleasure from your food choices. Sometimes your poor food selections can be attributed to social, cultural, and emotional issues. Poor food selection, poor stress management skills, and lack of activities are all behaviors that can attribute to weight gain. Another cause of weight gain can be attributed to the amount of time you are consuming food outside of your home. Many people, at some point in their life have used food as a coping mechanism. How often and to what extent you give in to external eating cues (parties, aroma, advertisements) usually has an impact on your weight gain. Food is socialy acceptable and can be used without indictment but the road to healthier eating can begin with pre-planning healthy meals and adjusting your caloric intake to meet your appropriate energy expenditure.

Throughout the years, dietitians and nutritionists have advocated weight loss through a balanced, energy controlled diet in conjunction with lifestyle changes to produce moderate consistent weight loss. Significant calorie restriction does produce rapid weight loss through loss of glycogen stores and possibly decreased caloric intake associated with the *"lack of choices"* in the restricted diet. In the mid 1970's, very low-calorie liquid diets (VLCLD), became commercially available, costs for such programs ranged from $250.00 to $3,000.00, depending on the weight loss desired. Meanwhile, low-calorie balanced diets were literally being packaged and sold to dieters, coupled with follow-up monitoring and counseling. Because patrons/participants in these programs were not apprised of the fact that weight loss wasn't permanent, criticism was pointed at the diet industry for not providing accurate information. (These programs did not inform the public about the rate of weight loss and how long participants were able to keep the weight off). In part due to these ommissions the Federal Trade Commission (FTC) stipulated weight loss companies to substantiate their weight loss claims in objective scientific studies, to state the average length of time customers maintained weight loss, and to include a disclaimer in their promotional information that many dieters find weight loss only temporary. Many commerical weight loss programs still exist in the new millenium but with significant more individualized offerings. Most programs now emphasize exercise and behavior modification as a critical component to total energy expenditure (weight loss/maintenance). Total energy expenditure correlates to physical activity, food digestion, and resting metabolism. Metabolism is the total sum of all vital processes by which energy and nutrients are made available to and used by your body.

*"**Behavior and genetics affect metabolic rates, not fad or restrictive diets alone**".* Fad and new diets pop up all the time claiming to have found the solution to weight loss, one book advocates eating meals high in protein, the next, low protein and still another will advocate a eating more complex carbohydrates or less sugar. If you are able to follow a restrictive diet and you are obtaining the results you desire, I applaud you, but the true bottom line is, if you consume more calories than your body is burning, no matter where the calories are coming from you are going to gain weight. Adopting Healthy Conscious Eating habits can combat this problem as opposed to restrictive dieting, which have been proven to be not effective for long-term weight loss and have been proven to be associated with lower metabolic rates. Thus when you return to your original eating habits you will regain the weight and possibly more.(A person who continues to diet and fast sporadically becomes metabolic efficient. This means that to maintain any weight after a drastic diet one has to eat less than another person with equal body weight who never lost weight because of the disproportional fat/lean ratio in the weight regain).

Before commiting to a restrictive commercial or medical weight loss program or a self-imposed total or modified fast make sure that you are armed with sound nutritional advice, a behavioral change plan, and/or advice for proper weight loss/maintenance. Most nutritional experts will agree that Americans consume more fat than is necessary for a balanced meal. Despite the recommended idea of 30 percent or less fat in your diet, Americans typically consume anywhere from 36 to 38 percent of their meals in fat and 40 percent of their meals as complex carbohydrates.

Complex carbohydrates are somewhat useful when attempting to lose weight simply because it requires your body to actually use calories (10% thermic effect) to convert the complex carbohydrates to glucose. Also eating complex carbohydrates in moderation can usually give you a feeling of fullness. You should also pay very close attention to your sugar intake when dieting. Excess sugar in your diet can result in weight gain immediately. Sugar is associated with your "good time" or "pleasure" foods and you must pay close attention to food labels because most sugars are hidden in the processing of convenience foods. (Sugars are hidden under names such as fructose, corn syrup, honey, sucrose, lactose, maltose, dextrose and mannitol). A good practice would be to substitute fresh or even frozen fruit for sugar cravings.

You should eat several small meals throughout the day in a consistent manner or daily routine. Breakfast should be eaten daily, followed by a snack (if desired), lunch should follow and then another snack (if needed). Dinner should be planned and eaten with the idea that you will soon be retiring for the evening. Listen to your body's physical response (internal cues) to hunger. Physical internal cues to hunger include minor headaches, fatigue, weakness or stomach rumbling. Avoid late evening or bed time snacking. A good way to avoid late night snacking would be to avoid taking your favorite foods or snacks out of the cupboards or refrigerator with the anticipation of eating them later as snacks. Leave them in the cupboards or refrigerator, you can always eat those foods in moderation at other times. Physical activity burns calories and keeps metabolism geared toward using food for energy instead of storing it as fat.

Your body relies on a specific caloric intake to carry out it's bodily functions (BMR). What this means is when you eat a certain amount of calories over a specific period of time you are giving your body a signal that this is the amount of calories that you need to carry out your vital bodily functions and your daily activities. If you exceed this amount on a continuous basis you then give your body a different signal that indicates you need more stored calories for later usage. For example, if your daily caloric intake is approximately 1,500 calories and you increase your caloric intake upwards to 2,500 calories once and awhile, this is acceptable (although not advisable). Periodically, you can overeat because what normally happens is your body will utilize the 1,500 calories as it normally would and then raise its metabolic rate to burn the excess 1,000 calories that you consumed. If you continue to intake upwards of 2,500 calories then you begin giving your body a different signal that indicates you now need more calories (energy) to carry-out your daily chores and daily vital bodily functions. As oppose to your body storing the 1,500 calories and raising its metabolic rate to burn the excess 1,000 calories, your body will now store the 2,500 calories for its anticipated later usage and when this expenditure does not happen you will have a weight gain over a period of time.

The time frame for weight gain/loss is different for everyone. Weight gain is predicated on metabolic rate, choice, and quantity of food. Eat food for energy from a variety of sources. Carbohydrates, fats and proteins should be eaten daily in proportion to your weight loss goals. A good rule of thumb to avoid loss of lean muscle mass is to intake protein from a wide variety of food choices such as beef, steaks, and chicken; also white breads or dinner rolls. Milk and poultry also provide protein. When meal planning for protein, keep in mind that foods are rated as complete or incomplete. Products such as pork, beef, fish, poultry, eggs, cheese, milk and other foods from animal sources are considered "complete" or "high quality" proteins because they provide all the essential amino acids. Remember to eat slowly allowing at least 20-30 meal to compete a meal and reduce your fat intake.

Fat percentage in your diet should not contain more than 10% of saturated fats. If you suffer from any coronary problems or your present lifestyle is completely sedentary you may want to limit your fat intake to even 7% or less of saturated fats in your diet. Remember, certain levels of fat are needed for your body's protection. Fat helps insulate your body from cold, provide cushion for your organs and is a good source of energy when utilized. Fat also adds flavor to food. Fat helps fuel your body at rest and at light activity levels. A certain percentage of the reserve energy you carry around is fat, which is a backup source of energy for your glycogen and glucose levels. Lipids or "fat" can be categorized as either saturated, unsaturated, or polyunsaturated. Foods are usually composed of both saturated and unsaturated fats. **Saturated fats** are those that contain large amounts of fatty acids and are usually found in animal flesh. You can usually find them as solids at room temperature and consist of things such as oils, soybean, sunflower and canola oils. Although fats provide 9 calories of energy per gram they are of little use at high levels of activity. Fats converts to energy usage only when mixed with carbohydrates at low intensity levels of activity unfortunately.

Several fat soluble vitamins ( B-1, K,E, A,D) are transported in the body by fat molecules and provide vitamins and minerals for your body. Vitamin B-1, (thiamin), is vital for the normal functioning of all body cells. It also helps the body break down carbohydrates, protein, and fat for energy. Sources: Lean cuts of pork, oysters, green peas, breads, cereal and whole grain. Vitamin A, is necessary for good eyesight, body tissue maintenance, growth and bone formation, vitamin A also aids your body in resistance to infection. Sources: liver, fish liver oils, whole or fortified milk, eggs, carrots and dark-green vegetables. Signs of Deficiency: Poor night vision or night blindness, loss of appetite, increased susceptibility to infection, and changes in your skin tone. The main function of vitamin K, is to regulate blood clotting. Sources of vitamin K, are milk, egg and margarine. A deficiency in vitamin K, is rare but can cause bleeding disorders because your blood will not be able to clot when needed. Vitamin E, acts as an antioxidant that stabilizes cell membranes and protects tissue throughout your body. It also protects fats and vitamin A, in your body from destruction. If inadequate, can lead to changes in your blood. Vitamin E, can be found in margarine, corn and peanut oils. Vitamin D, which is found in butter, and egg yolk, is valuable. Vitamin D, is essential in the formation and maintenance of bones and teeth by regulating the absorption and use of calcium and phosphorous. It also aids in the maintenance of a healthy muscle system. A deficiency can cause a weakening of your bones.

Another very important aspect of Healthy Conscious Eating is water. Water is a major nutrient for the human body. The body's water content remains relatively stable over time, any imbalance can be adjusted with appropriate intake. You should try to consume at least 64 ounces of filtered or bottled water daily. Add an additional eight ounces for every twenty-five pounds that you are overweight. Water makes up anywhere from 40%-60% of your body's mass and up to 75% of the weight of muscle and 50% of body fat. Remember, water is lost throughout the day by sweating and urine, this water needs to be replaced.

Your body's hypothalamus usually signals you when you are thirsty. The first sign of dehydration is thrist; if you are not taking in enough water, one sure sign will be lack of urine production. Water is a key part of any weight loss program. It is very necessary for helping the body remove fat and for general overall health. Water is also important for the following reasons:

A) Water helps to suppress your appetite.
B) Water assist your body in metabolizing stored fat.
C) Water aids in reducing sodium build-up.
D) Water helps to relieve constipation.
E) Water aids your body in removing waste and toxins.

You should realize that healthy conscious eating consist of variety, balance and moderation. To insure a balanced meal remember these few simple suggestions when meal planning. Food is the fuel/energy your body needs to keep functioning properly. What you eat supplies your body with the nutrients you need to maintain good health. *No single food or food group contains all the essential nutrients your body needs.* You must eat a variety of foods everyday to get all the nutrients essential to good health. Plan meals that are low in fat and use sugar in moderation. Although fat is considered bad, it does play an important role in your body. Fat helps to maintain healthy skin, insulates your body in cold temperatures and when called upon releases from your body as energy.

Pre-plan your meals and ***DRINK PLENTY OF WATER!***

Following is a sample pre-planned 1,500-calorie meal:

## BREAKFAST:

| ITEM: | AMOUNT: | CALORIES: | CARBOHYDRATES: | PROTEIN: | Saturated FAT: |
|---|---|---|---|---|---|
| Cereal | 1 cup | 220 | 49 | 4 | 0.0 |
| Milk | 1 cup | 102 | 12 | 8 | 2.0 |
| Banana | 1 medium | 105 | 27 | 1 | 0.0 |

### Snack
| | | | | | |
|---|---|---|---|---|---|
| Turkey | 3 ounces | 145 | 26 | 6 | 1.0 |
| Wheat bread | 2 slices | 148 | 0 | 0 | 0.0 |
| Mayonnaise | 3 tsp. | 22 | 1 | 1 | 0.0 |
| Lettuce | 1 cup | 7 | 1 | 0 | 0.0 |
| Water | 8 ounces | 0 | 0 | 0 | 0.0 |

### Lunch
| | | | | | |
|---|---|---|---|---|---|
| Veg. Soup | 1 cup | 72 | 12 | 2 | 0.0 |
| Chicken | 3 ounces | 140 | 0 | 26 | 1.0 |
| Spinach | ½ cup | 6 | 1 | 1 | 0.0 |
| Roll | 1 small | 85 | 14 | 2 | 0.0 |
| Water | 8 ounces | 0 | 0 | 0 | 0.0 |

### Snack
| | | | | | |
|---|---|---|---|---|---|
| Fresh Fruit | 1 piece | 72 | 19 | 1 | 0.0 |

## Dinner

| | | | | | |
|---|---|---|---|---|---|
| Strip Steak | 3 ounces | 176 | 0 | 24 | 3.0 |
| Wild Rice | ½ cup | 83 | 17 | 3 | 0.0 |
| Broccoli | ½ cup | 22 | 4 | 2 | 0.0 |
| Roll | 1 small | 85 | 14 | 2 | 0.0 |
| Water | 8 ounces | 0 | 0 | 0 | 0.0 |
| | | | | | |
| Totals | | 1,495 | 207 | 108 | 9.0 |

A delicate balance between energy intake and energy expenditure often is not maintained in sedentary individuals. This lack of precision in regulating food intake at the lower end of the physical activity spectrum may account for the creeping weight gain. Individuals who live an active lifestyle and practice Healthy Conscious Eating may eventually fall within a reactive zone in which food intake readily matches daily energy expenditure. You must maintain a certain level of fat which is really stored energy that you haven't burned off. Your body has a great capacity to hold this excess fat if you do not burn it off through your activity level. Remember your body has a great survival mechanism that allows you to store food/energy for periods of famine but in today's society you rarely, if at all, are faced with famine. Food is abundant and relatively inexpensive, thus you have excess intake that translates into additional body fat. It is strongly recommended that average body fat for women not exceed 25% and for men 20%.

To Calculate your body fat percentage use the equation below:

## Example:

| | |
|---|---|
| Female body weight: | 140 pounds x 25%=35 pounds (% body fat) |
| Male body weight: | 170 pounds x 20%=34 pounds (% body fat) |

Of course there are numerous other ways to test body fat percentage (refer to chapter 2), but for our purpose the calculation method above will suffice. It is imperative to understand body fat pecentages and its relationship to weight as well as body mass index.

### To calculate your body mass index (BMI), use the calculations below.

### Example:

A female who is 5'4 and weighs 145 lb., would calculate the BMI as follows:
145 lbs. /2.2=66 kilograms of weight.
5'4 ft. tall=64 inches in height.
64 inches in height x 0.0254=1.6 meters
1.6 meters x 1.6 meters=2.6 meters squared
66 kilograms / 2.6 meters=25.38 (BMI)

Let's Talk! After calculating your body fat percentage, resting metabolic rate, BMI and new caloric intake (See Appendix E), learn to like your body and become more physically active. Decide the approach that is best suited for you. Remember you are attempting to get motivated, so you should avoid goals that are out of your range, but your goals should not be so soft that you don't extract the benefits of your efforts. In the beginning, do not obsess with your weight and concentrate on improving your health.

The healthier you are the more active you can be. As your level of activity raises; the more weight you may eventually lose. Everyone has certain inner feelings about the weight that they feel most comfortable. Forget about weighing yourself for the first 5-6 weeks. Setting reasonable weight loss goals involves understanding that small to moderate weight loss over a prolonged period of time is more effective than regaining weight from a dramatic weight loss program. Weight loss of 10% -15% may be achieved through self-awareness, behavior modification, healthy conscious eating, increased activity levels and/or medication. Enjoy your newfound strategy and develop new habits with regards to your activity levels and healthy normal food consumption.

Normal food consumption does not mean restrictive eating or total liquid nourishment as meal replacements. Healthy conscious eating means being able to eat when you are physically hungry and continue eating until you are satisfied. Healthy Conscious Eating is being able to use some moderate constraints in your food selection to get the right food, but not being so restrictive that you miss out on pleasurable foods. Healthy conscious eating means giving yourself permission to eat; and to understand that eating is flexible. Eating will vary in response to your emotions, your schedule, your hunger, and sometimes due to your proximity to food. It is when you have adapted to an unhealthy eating syndrome that eating results in weight gain, poor health and adverse metabolic conditions.

# Chapter 5
## Cardiorespiratory Fitness

Let's Talk! The physiological, psychological, and social climate of today pressures everyone to be slim and fit. This has resulted in a heightened preoccupation and dissatisfaction with body image, which in turn, has led many people to try weight loss programs. Many overweight and obese individuals have had a long sedentary lifestyle and many have had poor experiences with increasing their activity levels.

Because of this, many overweight and/or obese individuals are at increased risk for orthopedic injury when starting a fitness program, and are encouraged to maintain low intensity activities for longer durations when initially increasing their activity levels. Incorporation of regular physical activities into your overall lifestyle can improve the chances of your weight loss success. The purpose of these activities are to promote strength, muscular endurance , flexibility, maintenance and improvement of lean muscle mass, and cardiorespiratory endurance.

Cardiorespiratory endurance is vital in regards to weight loss in obese individuals. Obese persons may suffer from respiratory insufficiency which causes them to be out of breath very quickly when increasing their activity levels. This is caused by a decreased in lung size, and the chest wall is very heavy and difficult to lift. At the same time, the demand for oxygen is greater. Enhancement of your cardiorespiratory system is necessary so that it allows you to perform the activities that you are attempting as well as everyday activities such as shopping, yard-work or climbing stairs. Your cardiorespiratory system includes the heart, lungs and circulatory system. The heart provides the impetus for blood flow. The average person's heart weighs less than a pound at rest, with an appropriate output of 1,400 gallons of blood daily.

The right side of the heart performs two important functions 1) it receives blood returning from all parts of the body and 2) it pumps blood to the lungs for aeration by way of pulmonary circulation. The left side of the heart also performs two important functions in that 1) it receives oxygenated blood from the lungs and 2) it pumps blood into the muscular aorta for distribution to the peripheral. When more oxygen is delivered to your cells you can become more efficient physically. Thus allowing minimal physical effort with maximal results. The more efficient the body becomes at utilizing oxygen the better it is able to cope with the stress of everyday physical activity.

Regular endurance activities produces improved cardiorespiratory

functioning and improved metabolism for better control of blood and body fats. During increased activity levels, your cardiorespiratory system must work harder to meet your body's increased demand for oxygen. We all agree that you have to breathe to stay alive and your lungs help you to breathe.

When you increase your activity levels you need more oxygen

delivered to your muscles and vital organs. You start breathing harder and more deeply during these times. Improved cardiorespiratory performance mproves the functioning of the gaseous exchange in your lungs.

This is important in that your lungs provide the separating surface between blood and surrounding gases. If the human body's oxygen supply depended only on diffusion through the skin this would be simple; but the body's ventilatory system plays a huge role in regulating the gaseous exchange of the body's external and internal environment. Air from the external environment is brought into your body by entering through your nose and mouth, it is adjusted to body temperature, filtered and humidified as it passes through your trachea. Before the air is taken into your lungs it passes through two bronchi that channels air into the lungs. This external air is now internal and eventually reaches your lungs through bronchioles and mixes with air in the alveolar ducts. Once inside the lungs, a gas exchange takes place; the lungs transfer oxygen from the air into the venous blood and move carbon dioxide from this blood into the alveolar chambers. This is very important; during each minute at rest, approximately 200 ml of carbon dioxide diffuses in the opposite direction. It is of primary importance that pulmonary functioning during rest and exercise is fairly constant and a favorable concentration of oxygen and carbon dioxide is maintained. During resting state each time you breathe and oxygen enters your body some of the oxygen is used by your red blood cells and transported to your heart. The oxygenated blood is pumped from your heart to your peripheral to organs and tissues that require it.

During increased activity levels, your cardiorespiratory system is required to work harder to get oxygenated blood to your peripheral. The increased demand for oxygen must be met before you are able to perform the activity that you are attempting. Once this demand is met you can now perform the activity or task with less exertion.

The adaptations that must occur (such as lowered exercise heart rate, lowered pulse, lowered blood pressure and increased oxygen consumption) for increased cardiorespiratory efficiency can be accomplished by stressing your body's cardiorespiratory system. For instance you may begin implementing your cardiorespiratory fitness regimen by walking 20-30 minutes a day at a leisurely, comfortable pace. Record the distance you have walked and remember the tempo that you were walking. When this pace becomes relatively easy to maintain, pick up the pace, and keep the same distance, recording the time it takes you to reach the original distance. Next increase your distance, but stay within the 20-30 minute time frame that you originally began with. Once this is achieved, revert back to your original time and distance and record how it corresponds to your perceived exertion level on a scale of 1 to 10, with the number 1 indicating minimal effort and the number 10 indicating total exhaustion. (It is important to monitor your exertion level so that you are not completely exhausted and risk injury). Continue this practice until you work up to 1 mile in 20 minutes .

Once this goal is attained you can begin to trim minutes off of your mile until you stress your body enough physically to burn the calories you are attempting to burn off. Remember the total oxygen cost of walking or running is linear, which means running or walking at 10 miles per hour requires about twice the energy per minute as running or walking at 5 miles per hour. In the first instance it takes maybe 6 –8 minutes and in the second instance it takes about 12-16 minutes, but the energy cost is the same. So, take your time and progressively build up to a comfortable pace. It is well established that active individuals have higher levels of cardiorespiratory fitness, and in controlled experimental trials, increase in activities resulted in increased fitness levels.

Another important aspect of cardiorespiratory fitness is improved metabolism. Your body's muscles does your body's work. Strength training activities usually increases the number of capillaries in your muscles causing hypertrophy of your muscle which can give you a chance for increased metabolism due to the larger muscle mass (Due to break down and repair of muscle tissue; Experts believe that as muscles are challenged by the resistance of weight, some of their tissue breaks down; as the muscle heals they gradually increase strength and size). By supplying your muscles with more oxygen and fuel they become more efficient. To burn fat during activity levels, you should incorporate longer periods of increased levels of activities as opposed to short high intensity levels. During high intensity activities, your body uses carbohydrates as its primary fuel source; this is roughly around the first 20 minutes. Fat is used as a secondary fuel source during high intensity activities but is used more efficiently to carry out the work of the body during periods of light activity, usually after 20 minutes of continuous activities. For most people, physcial activities performed at a steady pace, usually at 50% of your maximal oxygen consumption (considered to be a steady state of aerobic metabolism) will allow you to perform that activity for a prolonged period of time without the build-up of lactic acid (lactic acid build-up is the cause of the pain you feel when you are actively engaged in increased activities). When glycogen stores are depleted due to activity, lactic acid accumulates, causing your body to feel fatigued and requiring rest.

Remember during increased activities, your muscles use (carbohydrates) glycogen as their principle energy source; fat is a secondary fuel source, but is used more efficiently to carry out body processes during periods of rest and light activity. A person who is not fit will not have a sufficient supply of oxygen to their muscles to metabolize the amount of fuel needed for periods of intense activity. Glycogen will be used very rapidly and metabolic acids, particularly lactic acid will be produced. This lack of oxygen distribution allows lactic acid to build. Once it forms in the muscle, it rather quickly gets into the blood stream causing fatigue. But when sufficient oxygen is present, the formation pace of lactic acid is slowed.

At either low levels or high levels of activities, lactic acid accumulates. When activities are performed at high intensity levels, the demand for oxygen is greater and exceeds it rate of dispersion. Your body's ability to maintain a level of exertion for an extended period of time is a direct reflection of cardiorespiratory fitness. This is determined by your body's ability to utilize and distribute oxygen. So by increasing your oxygen consumption you will be able to sustain periods of activity longer.

If while participating in an aerobic and/or anaerobic activities and lactic acid stills accumulates it is best to stop the activity and allow your body to cool down. If you continue the activity it will only elevate your total metabolism to delay your recovery to steady state which results in you feeling fatigued longer from increased lactic acid build up in your body. When you engage in activities at an intensity greater than 60%, the steady state of aerobic metabolism cease and lactic acid formation exceeds its rate of removal, and blood lactate accumulates. As intensity increases, the level of lactic acid rises sharply causing fatigue.

Endurance activities also influences body chemistry by regulating energy balance. Energy balance and healthy conscious eating can lead to a healthy active lifestyle. Healthy conscious eating means eating a healthy, nutritious meal that provides all the nutrients the body need for essential functions. Even if you routinely prepare and eat a nutritiously balanced meal it can still be relatively high in calories, especially for a completely sedentary person. Healthy conscious eating coupled with an active lifestyle that includes increased activity levels aids in daily calorie expenditure so that healthy eating does not lead to weight gain. Long duration, moderately intense endurance activities and brief periods of more intense activities characterize fitness programs that best develop metabolic efficiency.

One of the best ways to protect lean body mass is to involve yourself in regular fitness activities that promote strength enhancement. We all know the basic principle of weight loss. Simply explained as burn more calories than you take in and increase your activity levels to burn stored fat. This can be accomplished with increased activity levels because what happens is your body will burn its own fat storage for energy. It is best to try and widen the gap between meals and increased physical activities as much as possible so that you burn the stored fat. When you incorporate healthy conscious eating into your particular lifestyle change program, remember that not all the weight you lose is in the form of fat. Diets that are extremely low in carbohydrates and proteins are likely to cause the loss of lean muscle mass as well as body fat.

Healthy Conscious Eating and increased activity levels can prevent loss of lean muscle mass and are two vital components to weight loss. Increasing your activity levels is a great escape from the craziness of everyday life. Increased activity levels can reduce anxiety and tension; due to the diverted reduced muscle tension that occurs with regular participation in high calorie/energy burning activities. Positive increased activity levels helps you to achieve balance. No one part of your body can be consistently overused (like your brain), without harming in some way another or other parts of your body. We, as a society, have become almost completely sedentary neglecting the body's physiological need to be active. A sedentary lifestyle creates adverse physiological conditions within your body. Diverse activities can assist in diverting some of your thoughts, it gives your mind a chance to rest and allows you to remain active. By increasing your activity levels, the once thought impossible can become possible.

Cardiorepsiratory fitness has an impact on the levels of fat in the blood also. High concentrations of blood fats like cholesterol and

triglycerides are linked to heart disease mainly because they contribute to the formation of fatty deposits within the arteries that supply blood to your heart. If your arteries become clogged or even blocked, a heart attack or stroke can occur.

Cholesterol is carried through your body in blood by lipoproteins and they are classified as Low Density Lipoproteins (LDL), or High Density Lipoproteins (HDL), according to their size and density. The Low Density Lipoprotein (LDL), usually referred to as the bad ones because they carry cholesterol from your liver to parts of your body that needs them. Problems can occur when LDL carry more cholesterol than is needed by your body and the excess is deposited into your blood vessels and accumulates. When low density lipoproteins accumulates on your arterial walls they trigger the formation and build up of white blood cells which then form a fatty substance known as plaque. As plaque builds up, your arterial walls constrict reducing your blood flow which is a major contributor to coronary heart disease. High Density Lipoproteins (HDL), considered the good guys, carry unused cholesterol from your body and walls of your arteries back to your liver for recycling.

High density lipoproteins are important for that reason. High levels of high density lipoproteins (above 45 mg/dl) appears to protect your arteries from plaque buildup. A number of studies have demonstrated that low density lipoprotein levels (160 mg/dl) and total cholesterol levels of below 200 mg/dl are optimal. High levels of high density lipoproteins are as important as low levels of low density lipoproteins. Also one should note that cholesterol levels are not exact; what is important to realize is the ratio of low density lipoprotein to high density lipoprotein (a desirable ratio would be 3.5 (LDL) to 1 (HDL).

# Chapter 6
# Increasing Muscular
# Strength & Endurance

The unequivocal acceptance of the notion that thinness equals beauty, health, and fitness can sometimes create obstacles for large people who want to improve their health status through lifestyle changes.

Let's Talk! As Americans we seldom walk when we can ride. We prefer elevators and escalators to stairs. A majority of people have jobs that require sitting during most of the workday and when they are off from work they are to busy to engage in physical activities. In essence, they are leading a somewhat sedentary lifestyle. By not adhering to an active lifestyle and consuming high-fat, high caloric foods, you can, and most likely have become caloric efficient.

Adapting to a active lifestyle can be thought of as a system of choice or attitude. It means traveling on foot when possible and safe as opposed to riding in vehicles. It means taking the stairs when feasible as opposed to using the elevator. It means finding ways to increase your energy expenditure while decreasing your caloric intake. It means developing healthy ways of dealing with stress, boredom, fatigue, and loniless that do not involve food. It means monitoring your blood pressure and cholesterol levels, and your overall health status in relation to your weight.

Some guidelines to follow are listed below.

Goal:       Increase caloric expenditure.
Mode:       First choice is walking; Alternative modes; include stair climbing, cycling, and water exercises.

Intensity:    Should be at the low end of target heart rate, i.e., 50% to 60% of maximum oxygen consumption.

Duration:    Sufficient to cause expenditure of 200 to 300 kcal/session.

Frequency:    Should be minimum of three times a week.

Taken from The American College of Sports Medicine guidelines for exercise prescription for obesity reduction and weight management:

The guidelines also offer the following exercise prescriptions for the obese:

* Avoid stress on joints.
* Choose a setting that minimizes social stigma.
* Monitor muscle soreness and othopaedic problems.

Because obese individuals are at an increased relative risk for orthopedic injuries, most individuals are encouraged to maintain lower intensities and longer durations of increased activities in order to meet the energy expenditure goal of 200 to 300 kcal/session. Many obese individuals have had a long sedentary lifestyle and many have had poor experiences with increasing their activity levels in the past. In addition to obtaining medical clearance prior to increasing your activity levels, ideally the obese should begin their programs under the guidance of a professional (optional). Under such supervision, past negative experiences can be overcome and current strengths and interest can be emphasized.

The benefits of increased activity levels and strength training include not only more **calorie expenditure**, but also **low cholesterol levels,** and **greater muscle mass** (which uses more calories for fuel than fat cells do). Since muscle metabolizes three times quicker than fat, even when resting, it is beneficial to engage in strength training activities. Strength training increases muscles and connective tissue size and density by enlarging cells, or "building" muscles. Larger muscles and connective tissues aid in long term weight control by increasing your metabolism. Strength training activities also enhances the ability of your body's muscles to produce extreme amounts of force in a short period of time when called upon for easy and coordinated daily activities such as climbing stairs, gardening, carrying groceries, and walking. The more you ask of your body the more you will get from it! Your body will adapt to the greater demands that are placed upon it (due to repeated use of specific muscles).

The stronger you are, the less likely you are to suffer injuries that keep you from staying active and having fun. Prior to engaging in a strength training, aerobic/anaerobic comprehensive program for weight loss you must first familiarize yourself with two key terms 1) specificity, which means performing specific activities for specific results; and 2) progressive overload, which means stressing the body to the point where changes occur. These factors can be determined by addressing frequency, duration and intensity. Frequency dictates that you should engage in your specific work out a minimal of three times a week. You do not necessarily have to purchase a membership at a private or commercial fitness center or hire a personal trainer to obtain a work-out. You can simply increase your present activity levels and incorporate a few new activities in all aspects of your daily life. Membership to a gym or fitness center does give you more of a variety, options and a greater challenge, but remember you are your own coach, take charge of your life and regain your health by adhering to a successful weight loss and weight management program that incorporates increased aerobic and anaerobic activities, provide the necessary nutrients your body needs, and fits into your lifestyle.

A good beginning is to target aerobic activities such as walking, jogging, or running that require you to expend (180-700 calories per 30 minute session). Walking knows no boundaries. You do it everyday, so few people are excluded from engaging in this activity. Walking at a moderate pace is a popular fitness activity, doesn't require a lot of financial investment and can be just as effective as other fitness activities. Any style of walking is okay when you are just beginning, but once you have worked up to 1.0 mile in 30 minutes, it is time to increase the pace and decrease the time. Increase the pace by taking shorter quicker steps.

The initial objectives are to gain the benefits of the increased activity level, enhance performance and burn calories, so the longer you sustain an elevated heart rate, the more fat you can burn. If you walk at a moderate pace for 25 minutes you will essentially have twenty-five minutes of continuous burned calories. It is advisable if you have been sedentary for a while to work out initially at a very low intensity for approximately 10-15 minutes and gradually build up to longer durations and higher intensity. This will allow you to burn more calories from your fat substrate while enhancing your fitness level. Remember to walk with your head up, shoulders relaxed, stomach pulled in, and rear muscles tight . Walking with your head down can strain your back and shoulders and interfere with your breathing.

Walking at a low intensity level burns more fat than if done at a higher intensity, places less stress on your body, and if done fast and far enough (5-10 miles per hour for approximately 45-60 minutes) can be just effective as running or jogging. Higher intensity levels of walking (i.e. speedwalking) are better for building strength in your arms and torso and streamlining flabby thighs (pear shape). If you prefer to begin your weight loss, fitness program by running instead of walking, running burns more calories per minute than many other sports and is considered one of the best aerobic exercises. Running is certainly one way to push your pulse into your target heart zone and keeping it there for 30 minutes or more. When beginning, try to run every other day, allowing six to eight weeks to build up to a 30-minute sustain run.

Beware running places intense stress on your joints; about three of four times your body weight with every bouncing step, (about 3,000 steps every 20 minutes). Many individuals make the mistake of running too fast, too far, too soon, which can cause injury. A healthy running program will vary between hard days and easy days. Train for endurance first and worry about speed later. Running strengthens your legs, helps develop your endurance, ease tension, boost your energy, and burns 585-700 calories an hour, depending on your speed and size. It doesn't do much for your upper body, though, so consider adding a strength training program with your running program (if you enjoy running, as opposed to walking), for a comprehensive weight maintenance plan.

Regardless, whether you opt for walking, jogging, running or a combination of the three invest in a pair of quality tennis shoes, with good support and room in the toe area that support your feet, and provides good ankle support that aids in preventing injury. While progressing through your comprehensive fitness plan, remember the amount of overload is very important. Minimal activities will not have a great effect on your fitness level; and too much overload, too soon may cause injury. If injury occurs stop the activity immediately. When pain occurs due to injury, it is a signal, a protective measure to guard your body from further damage or action that might cause further harm.

Barring injury you should progress with the progressive overload and specificity and continue working diligently. External results and physical adaptations should appear around the 6th-8th week of training. Prior to this all of the necessary adaptations ( i.e., muscular hypertrophy, increased oxygen consumption)are ocurring internally.

The goal of fitness training is to bring about long-term changes and efficiency in your body's performance and functioning. Remember to train your body the way you want your body to respond. Stress your body so that the adaptations that occur are the adapatations you desire. For instance do not work out with heavy weights if you do not want a heavy muscular appearance. Instead work out with lighter weights at higher intensities and duration. Do not work on speed while jogging, if your purpose for jogging is to lose weight, because the longer the jog and sustained heart rate the better it is for weight loss.

Through healthy conscious eating, a comprehensive fitness program that encompass strength training, aerobic, and anaerobic activities coupled with regular monitoring of your body fat you can achieve a healthy body weight. To achieve the best results from your time and efforts, you should design your strength and conditioning program to fit into your daily lifestyle and it allows you to achieve maximal results and have low risk of injury to you. As previously stated, your muscles will get stronger if you make them work. Resistance training is usually a good way to enhance your muscular strength and endurance. Machines or free weights are great for building strength safely and effectively. Free weights are usually a good start for someone who is just beginning a strength program if you learn the proper way to lift and avoid overexerting yourself. The initial weight usage can be determined by lifting a pre-determined weight (guess at what you can lift once without straining), after that one repetition lift is used to determine beginning weight you can now begin your strength training program.

Weight machines are less risky and easier to control, but are usually not a practical option for most because of cost. If you are able to purchase exercise equipment, it can be a good investment for your health and enjoyment. Weight machines are safe, convenient, and after the initial familiarity phase, can become easy to use. Machines can make it easier to keep track of your workout, increase intensity, and work specific muscle groups. Although both free weights and weight machines eventually give you the same results, free weights does require more care, greater concentration and balance. Choose weights based on your current fitness level and set goals. If you desire to build muscle mass quickly, you should increase your activity weights as rapidly as possible without risking injury. If your goal is to build endurance, mainly as opposed to bulk, then you should utilize comfortable weights with more repetitions.

Your fitness program should be tailored to incorporate both strength and endurance. It is advisable to warm up prior to the weight lifting session by stretching, walking or lifting a very light weight for a few moments to give your body time to prepare for your more intense weight training activities. To cool down you should relax for several minutes or repeat a stretching routine. Remember to stop in between sets to allow your muscles a brief period of rest. (Whether you choose free weights or machines, the first few weeks of your strength-training program should be devoted to learning the machine and learning the techniques of each activity you choose to implement into your fitness program). You should incorporate weight training into your fitness routine between two and four days per week to allow for muscle mass development to remain. Allow your muscles to rest the days you are not strength training to avoid over usage (You shouldn't experience pain when strength training but you should expect to feel some muscle soreness the next day).

As an alternative to free weights and weight machines some individuals choose to develop increased muscular strength and endurance using isokinetic or isometric activities. These type of activities involves exerting force at a constant speed against an equal force exerted by a special strength-training machine. The machines provide resistance to the joints a different ranges of motion. Some individuals prefer isometric activities that require no equipment at all. This type of activity builds muscle strength rapidly while burning fat, and is useful to individuals who are recovering from things such as work injuries, surgical interventions for weight loss or for people who have been sedentary for quite some time. If you choose this type of strength building routine it is very important to remember to achieve maximal results you must perform the activities at different angles utilizing different parts of your body (e.g., walking, jogging, calisthenics).

Thirdly, increasing your activity levels can cause you to feel better, physically and mentally. You should want a strong, healthy attractive body. You should realize that to acquire this for more than a few months out of a year will require lifelong changes in your activity levels and eating habits. Why do people let their programs fizzle out? There are many reasons, however, the main underlying reason is negative attitude.

When you begin viewing your program as a negative chore, it soon becomes one. Most of us find time to do the things we enjoy. People who learn to enjoy the rewards of physical activity have the same kind of enthusiasm for their workouts as those individuals who enjoy shopping, attending or viewing sporting events and to some degree, can compare with the party goers who look forward to happy hour or dining out on Friday nights.

One of the hardest parts of starting a program, and maintaining it, is finding the time on a regular basis. The spare minutes for a walk, run or weight lifting session just aren't there. If you view physical activity as punishment for being overweight that you have to tolerate, your program will be hard to continue. You can turn this attitude around by replacing negative self-talk with positive self-talk. Most of us carry on a silent conversation with ourselves on a daily basis. These conversations can actually improve or hamper your motivation throughout the day. Understanding what these thoughts are and how they affect you can be instrumental in replacing negative self-talk with postitie self-talk and assisting you in committing to increasing your physical activity levels.

Self-talk is a self-fulfilling prophecy, when your self-talk is positive, the results can be in your favor. When your self-talk is negative, you are not giving yourself a chance and your results may be negative. You should think of increasing your activities as the time of day you have for yourself. Remind yourself that diverse activities helps you to relax tense muscles and relieves stress. Focus on the good feelings you get after a workout.

Remember to train regularly, because adaptations are reversible and you must not give your body time to revert back to its former level. Understand that it is a gradual progression to a healthier lifestyle and weight maintenance. It does not happen over night and it does not come without healthy conscious eating, effort, understanding, work, education, and behavioral changes. TRAIN YOUR BODY AND MIND!

# Chapter 7
# Understanding Stress

What exactly is stress? Let's Talk! Stress is a word that most people blurt out when things are not going well and their body is drained of energy and their thinking becomes unclear. How well do you manage your stress? How committed are you to your professional life, social life and hobbies? Are you a risk taker, a person who believes that the higher the risk, the greater the reward? Whether stress is experienced as a good thing or bad thing depends largely on the individual and the situation.

Regardless to your perception of a given situation stress is present in most instances and can be defined as your body's total biological response to a stressor. Stress is inevitable and will not go away, but it can be managed. Stress can be short-term (acute), or long-term (chronic); Good or bad. It's when there are too many good and bad challenges confronting you at once and you lose your ability to judge them appropriately, the stressors in your life causes you distress. Everyday hassles can cause as much stress as large unexpected events. Worries such as financial, arguments and/or disputes, a break-up or divorce, a death in the family, losing a job or even buying a home can cause an unbelievable amount of stress to an individual. Stress is unavoidable, but that doesn't mean it's unmanageable. A walk around the block or a vigourous workout, a nutritious meal, and/or a good night's sleep will usually give you the energy and strength to face another day. However, taking these simple steps may not help when occasional stress turns into chronic stress.

***Chronic Stress*** cracks your emotional foundation making you angry, apathetic, irritable, anxious or even depressed. You may quit eating altogether or eat too much. You may find it hard to concentrate or you may start smoking. Too much stress may even make you more accident prone, lead to alcohol or drug abuse and affect your body's immune system, thus increasing vulnerability to diseases. (Some studies suggest that acute stress actually boost your immune system. If stress becomes chronic however, this hypersensitive immune response is dull making you more vulnerable to colds, eczema and headaches).

Most people view stressors as negative , such as job deadlines, financial worries, or traffic jams. The physiological changes your body undergoes during the stress response are not recognized or ignored by most; but most people can identify with the tense muscles, headaches or stomachaches, during, before, or after a stressful event.

Stressors can be positive as well as negative. Planning a wedding, having a baby or winning a million dollar lottery prize are positive things that can also induce the physiological stress response. Your physiological response to stress is a survival mechanism that has remained unchanged for thousands of years and is triggered each time you experience a stressful event.

These physiological changes are called your "fight-or-flight" response survival mechanism, which has remained unchanged for thousands of years. This survival mechanism aided prehistoric man's survival by helping him to run away from danger faster or to fight harder and is a part of your biological inheritance. Following a threat or perceived threat your hypothalamic pituitary adrenal gland releases catecholamines known as dopamine, norepinephrine (brake), and epinephrine (gas), these chemicals serve as messengers to your brain. The catecholamines triggers your emotional response to stress and stores the response in your memory. The catecholamines also suppress activity in your brain that alters your short term-memory, concentration and rational thought. This is necessary to allow you to react to the actual or perceived danger (stresor) quickly (fight-or-flight).

In prehistoric man this mechanism allowed him to recall large animals that were a previous threat and of danger to him, and enabled him to either fight harder or flee the imminent danger (while recalling what happened during the last encounter). Modern day stressors are not of that magnitude and detriment yet, the same physiological response is triggered each time you experience a stressor.

Your body cannot distinguish between a positive or a negative stressor and responds to it (good or bad) in the same way. When you experience a situation as stressful your body reacts to the situation, independent of conscious thought by preparing your body to take physical action (fit-or-flight). Hormones, like adrenalin surge. Your hearing and vision become more acute, your heartbeat increases, your blood pressure increases, your blood sugar level rises to boost energy to your muscles and brain, and you begin to perspire in order to cool you down while endorphins are released in order to relive pain in case you are injured.

Managed and controllable stress can provide interest and excitement for some individuals and can even motivate some individuals (deadlines, goals, appointments) to greater achievements, where a lack of deadlines (stress), and goals (stress), can lead to boredom and depression for others. In modern times this physiological response inappropriately occurs because it is triggered without conscious thought (modern day stressors are different; therefore the response when repeated continuously can cause fatigue and dysfunction, hindering your ability to handle complex social or intellectual tasks and behaviors). When normal function is disrupted by a stressor your body will attempt to restore itself back to homeostatis by calming your body down, slowing heart rate and breathing to a normal steady state. This process utilizes a great deal of energy and can cause you to feel fatigued at the end of a day. Your body will resist change and will strive at all cost to return to normality (homeostatis).

Although everyone responds physiologically to stress in the same way, humans differ differently in their emotional and behavioral responses to stress. Some individuals may present confident and relaxed, while others may panic and worry about the same stressor that is present to both. Coping skills with regards to emotional responses to stress can be helpful in dealing with stressful situations. Temperament, life perceptions & experiences as well as beliefs and ideas aid in stress management and individual variations.

Behavioral responses to stress; such as laughing, crying, talking and/or physical activity can be comforting and therapeutic. Stress is like room temperature if it's not in the proper balance for you, functioning becomes difficult. Remember stress can be perceived as both good and bad. Regardless of the type of stress you are experiencing, your body needs to have periods of rest. During periods of rest you allow your body to recover from the physiological responses it has undergone.

Take a brief moment to answer the questions on the following page and grade yourself on your current stress level and awareness.

_____ 1. I am often angry .
_____ 2. I believe in treating others fairly.
_____ 3. You create your own breaks in life.
_____ 4. I speak up for what I believe is right.
_____ 5. I am honest about my feelings.
_____ 6. Getting out of bed in the morning is hard for me.
_____ 7. I've been known to break things when I am angry.
_____ 8. I sometimes feel like hitting people.
_____ 9. I often curse when things go wrong.
_____ 10. I am easily frustrated in traffic.
_____ 11. I am furious when I am embarrased.
_____ 12. I have the freedom I want.
_____ 13. It seems like I am arguing a lot.

_____     14. I know what is important in my life.
_____     15. I use my time wisely.

Score 0 if the statement is definitely not true for you; 1 if it is usually not true; 2 if it is somewhat true; 3 if it is definitely true. Now total your score, if your score is above 30, you have good stress management skills, if your score is between 29-20, you have a good start and understanding of what it may require to manage your stress. Below 20 you are in danger of repeating the stress response continuously. Reach out for help and begin increasing your activity levels along with healthy conscious eating, and implementing a behavioral change process.

Stress is here to stay. The question is not how to avoid stress, but rather how to cope wIth it. High levels of stress can make it difficult to have balance in your life. When you no longer have balance in your life, your focus is no longer clear. One reason for the general confusion about stress is that the physiological and emotional reactions are defined in different ways. Stress is a normal part of life, but serious stress that depresses your mood or ruins your ability to experience joy may be the result of an anxiety disorder or depression. So how do you gain control?

Let's Talk! People who effectively manage the stress in their lives have several things in common. They consider life a challenge, not a series of hassles. They have a mission or purpose in life and are committed to fulfilling that mission. They do not feel victimized by life, but believe that even when they experience temporary setbacks, they have control over their lives. The important components of successful lifestyle management are knowledge, and changing attitude and the belief that you have more control over the things that happen in your life. If you believe you will succeed and if you recognize and accept the fact that you are in charge of your life not your friends or parents, not your genes, not even circumstances beyond your control, then you are well on your way to succeeding in a weight loss program, whether commercial or self-imposed.

Most behaviors are habits that have been learned. They may be deeply ingrained, long standing habits, but they are still habits. You can unlearn them the same way you learned them. The key is to approach them in a systematic way. Behavioral self-management. Behavioral change is important in managing stress. Stress cannot be eliminated only managed, and a good way to begin reducing and managing stress is to restructure your priorities and identifying stressors in your life. Take an inventory of your daily life. Start a journal/diary listing the things that puts a strain on your energy and time. Pay close attention to the events that triggers your emotional responses such as anger and/or anxiety. Identifying these factors can help identify the things in your life that you may want to change. By setting goals you can begin to change the things you can and develop a better lifestyle for things that you cannot change.

Life is filled with stressful events, both good and bad. Your body's stress response is like a rocket ship. Although all systems are stable on its launching pad, when it takes off; all systems are go! When your stress response is activated, all systems are go! This survival mechanism was essential in primative times and can be activated by modern day stressors. Your fight-or-flight response allows you to react quickly if needed but because modern day stressors are different your stress response when continuously activated can hinder your ability to handle complex social or intellectual situations if not given the proper outlet.

Stress can diminish your quality of life by reducing your feelings of pleasure and accomplishments, and chronic stress with poor management may result in anxiety disorders or depression addictions.

# Chapter 8
# The Psychological Aspects of Healthy Conscious Eating!

Let's Talk about the social and psychosocial aspects of healthy conscious eating, and what happens when you sabotage your own weight loss efforts. To begin, ask yourself who do you think is more susceptible to unconscious eating, the overweight or underweight? These are important factors because many people cannot gain control of their eating behaviors until they realize there are unconscious and/or subconscious reasons for eating. Individuals who have struggled with weight throughout their lives are usually aware that there are unconscious and subconscious forces which can undermine otherwise healthy eating; but how do you address those forces.

The complex social and psychosocial forces one must face can be both cause and effect of an unhealthy eating regimen. The cause and effect get lost overtime, as an unhealthy eating regimen becomes habit. That is what we are talking about, is it not? Unhealthy eating becomes a sustained response to emotions often cued by your social interactions with your primary groups(s), like family, church, etc. Psychologically, healthy conscious eating has a unique meaning for individuals trying to lose weight. In a nutshell, it means getting to know yourself through self-exploration. Specifically, it means gathering an honest appraisal of what food means to you individually, as a family and culturally.

Let's Talk! No one becomes overweight or obese because they want to! People become overweight and/or obese, and even morbidly obese because they eat too much compared to the amount of exercise and activity that comprise their daily lives. But **no one** wants, nor deserves the ridicule, abuse and discrimination that comes with being FATTER than their friends, family and everyone else in their environment. So why do we let ourselves become overweight? The answer is that we become overweight inspite of our best attempts not to do so because there are subconscious and even unconscious forces which drives us to eat even when we are not hungry. Our eating patterns are influenced by thoughts, feelings, desires, social events occurring in our environment, **as well as** our body's physiological needs such as hunger.

Although each of us has genetic tendencies to either be heavy (efficient depositor of energy as fat) or thin (inefficient at storing fat for later energy needs) our ultimate body shape has been influenced not only by our genes but also by how we respond to other stimuli. These other stimuli that influence our eating habits include external cues (advertising, the smell of food, the time we usually eat), social interactions (meeting friends where food is served), our subconscious state of mind (we are bored, angry, lonely or hurt) and our brain's unconscious forces which drives our behavior without us even appreciating it.

I know what you are probably thinking. This is just another diet book right? Well, it may be perceived by some to be another diet book because we are suggesting ways to improve your relationship with food. We understand that throughout a person's life food may assume a personal meaning that reaches far beyond hunger. Food makes people feel good, and fatty foods can make people feel very good. Because of this, food has much more than just biological meaning to people, for some people, it's a friend, for some people, it's a best friend, and for some people it's an only friend. So, on the other hand, if we can help you view your friend (food) in a new way, we may help to improve your relationship with food.

Understand that your friend (food) may have over stayed his/her welcome in many instances, and you can find other ways to feel better and establish other relationships. Asking food not to be so important to you "*all the time*" may be too difficult or plain impossible. But it is possible to develop more self-awareness and use that awareness to aid in your efforts to not use food to treat or pacify many of your emotions.

One of the most troubling influences we see in our everyday practice is the consequences of early sexual abuse. Although childhood sexual abuse is not a leading cause of obesity in children, when abuse has occurred, one of the most frequent unconscious responses is to eat and build bulk to have more physical power and also to become less attractive so that the sexual abuse will stop. This type of response does not stay in the conscious mind, however, because it is to painful and overwhelming. If it stayed in your conscious; fulltime depression and even suicidal ideation might result. Instead, it becomes buried in the subconscious almost immediately and soon becomes buried even deeper in the brain, in the limbic system, the unconscious. This defensive response maybe necessary for life to continue and is the reason that many adults with terrible childhood experiences do not remember them except in dreams, flashbacks or through therapeutic efforts to understand the causes of underlying behaviors with a professional such as a psychologist or psychiatrist.

Other less frightening childhood experiences also can lead to subconscious and unconcious forces influencing our daily habits and activities. Children are not always sophisticated enough to understand that they cannot control their environment and often develop deep feelings of guilt if their parents divorce (because they assume it was their fault). Sometimes a sibling dies or a child has an overreaction to more common events such as terror if left with strangers (even at school or day care) that have to do with the body's response to abandonment, or fears of not being loved.

If someone has had one of these terrible childhood experiences that has influenced their subconcious and unconscious behavior patterns, a book like this will not help them lose weight. If obesity has developed in part, as a protective response (even though obesity by itself will not be protection), any decrease in weight will cause individuals with these influences to become anxious and to sabotage their weight loss efforts when these significant psychological problems are involved, professional counseling with a psychotherapist is needed to address these issues before there can be any hope that someone can lose weight.

If you are aware that you have had an experience that still causes bad dreams or terror, or if you find yourself deliberately sabotaging your weight loss efforts, you need to consult a psychotherapist to discuss these feelings with them. Many other common experiences we can all relate to influence our eating behaviors in subconcious and unconscious ways. Most of us know that almost all parents try to pacify a crying infant by feeding them. A baby who is angry or afraid can often receive attention and comfort from being held and breast fed or even bottle fed because their "needs" are being met, even if the need being met was not hunger. This pattern persists and is re-enforced when we give toddlers candy or "sweets" like a cookie or an ice cream cone when they become "upset" rather than hungry. The receiving of food is perceived as an expression of the love rendered by the parents, relatives, or friends. A natural extension of this, is for us to treat our comfortable emotions by giving ourselves a food "treat" because in our subconcious/unconscious the brain receives this unneeded food as a partial response to an unmet need. Some of our patients understand they eat to treat their loneliness, boredom, guilt, anger, fear of abandonment (emotional eating) but at least a third of our patients are not in touch enough with their feelings to release this at a conscious level.

Whether it is unconscious or conscious, emotional eating is a behavior that is part of an eating pattern that is unhealthy and leads to the development of obesity. Our goal with this book is to help you develop "Healthy Conscious Eating" habits. This can only be done if you are willing to begin to define **"WHY"** you are eating. To get in touch with your emotions everytime you eat. Only then can you begin to make connections which will help you break destructive habits such as unhealthy eating because you are bored,anxious or stressed. If you can appreciate that you are bored, you can lose weight by telephoning a friend, or a relative, reading a good book, leaving the house to work in the garden, or go shopping rather than going into the kitchen and preapring a meal or snack. In chapter 2 we suggest that you keep a FOOD RECORD (DIARY), where you record every item you eat for several days, where you ate the item, and what you felt like when you decided to eat that item. This exercise is designed to initiate self-awareness with regards to your eating behavior and feelings; in other words to make you more aware of destructive behaviors! If you are "NOT" starving or at least very hungry, why are you searching for food? If your spouse, or your mother, or your boss made you angry; try writing them a memo or a letter (Even though you may never give this note to them), instead of eating a candy bar or drinking a high calorie drink to "soothe" yourself. This attitude change is the start of your successful weight loss program.

If someone hurts your feelings, when feasible take off on a walk or a drive in your car (CAUTION: NEVER DRIVE WHEN YOU ARE SO ANGRY THAT IT INTERFERES WITH YOUR SENSES AND/OR REFLEXES) or put on your favorite music while you think about how you should respond in the long run. Develop coping skills for this type of stimuli rather than searching for your favorite foods or snacks (comfort food). You will not always be successful at these choices but the very act of having to write down a food choice and the emotion that goes with it gives you time to think about this choice. It gives you an opportunity to stop bad habits while developing strategies to replace them with more healthy responses.

Healthy Conscious Eating!

We also emphasize tat you must learn to associate eating food with whether or not you are hungry and your boy's response to this hunger. To do this, get in touch with your emotional/physiological response to food. When you are trying to decrease your unnecessary eating and developing Healthy conscious Eating habits you need to develop your new relationship with food by paying attention to it. In earlier chapters of this book we suggest that you eat slowly, chewing each mouthful to get its full flavor and take time between each mouthful to give your body time to respond to the amount you have eaten. Consider your food diary part of your new relationship with food and record the amounts and the types of foods you choose. Take the time to know the caloric content of the food by reading the label on the package or looking up the number of calories in a reference book. Start with a smaller amount of food than you would usually eat and eat more only if you really need too. Or, you can order or prepare the usual amount of food and eat only half initially (give yourself a chance to be full/satisfied on less food), if you are still physically hungry you can eat the rest at a slower pace until satiety.

Make this your social time with your food rather than a social time with others. Too often, we make poor choices eating in social situations such as parties, school/church/religious meetings, sports events or work events. While you are learning to change your eating habits it is best to stay away from any event connected to food and socializing. At these events, If you must go to one of these functions while trying to lose weight, eat by yourself or before you go satisfy your hunger; but remember to convince yourself you will not eat or drink alcohol while at the event, it is too hard to keep track of your food intake because other activities are occupying your attention to know if you are eating to satisfy hunger, or simply eating because of external cues (aroma; sight; smell).

As you get more control over your "destructive" and/or "BAD" eating habits and adapt to a Healthy Conscious Eating lifestyle you can learn to enjoy these events without overeating. However, you have to have a conscious plan first. You have to choose ahead of time what items of food you will eat (i.e. vegetable based salad items rather than hot dogs or potatoe chips), when during the event you will eat (i.e. after you have talked with the people you want to see and focus your attention on), and use portion control before you start to eat (use the smallest plate or limit your trips to places where food is displayed). You still need to pay attention to the food you eat while eating. At one of these events. You need to get away from the crowd or **at least** be with uninteresting people that you can partially ignore so you have the ability to also listen to what your body is telling you. Once you stop eating, DO NOT restart especially for deserts unless this will be your only item. It is also important to realize that when you eat around other people, you are giving these people a chance to sabotage your Healthy Conscious Eating. Unfortunately, our society has trained all of us to enjoy the act of destroying our family and neighbors efforts to control their eating, it is one of our favorite national past-times.

Again, there are conscious and unconscious reasons we try to sabotage each other, but your goal is not to put yourself at risk. Never tell others your eating plans and learn to tell others you are not feeling well and are afraid of being sick (most people will not want you to vomit in front of them; but a few disturbed individuals will even obtain entertainment from pushing you to eat in this situation. Most efforts to sabotage your efforts to control your eating are caused by the need for those around you to feel superior, more in control of their lives than you are of yours.

Sometimes a family member or friend wants to see you happy, but still have resistance to decision to change your approach to food and attempt to persuade you to agree with their approach to food (i.e. when you eat my food, you let me know that you appreciate the time I spent preparing this meal/event). More often, most people around you, do not want you to change your weight because you then upset the status quo. If they are thinner than you they do not want you challenging their perceived superior position. If they are heavier than you, they view your commitment to becoming healthier as a condemnation of their lifestyle. The easiest way to avoid these conflicts are to avoid the event or avoid eating at the event even if it means pretending that you do not feel well (when you are obese you can honestly say you do not feel well and then protect your privacy by not telling the others **EXACTLY** why you do not feel well!)

If it is a family Thanksgiving dinner or some other event that cannot be missed then other previously mentioned strategies must be developed. The easiest strategy is often a combination of decreasing your eating and increasing your activity! **Get involved in activities that allow you to stay active. Get up from the table, take a walk even if there is no functional reason to move. Change the nature of the experience in a positive way for yourself.**

### Surgical Intervention for Weight Loss:

Everyone have heard the shouts, "I've had it with diets; I can't lose weight on a diet; diets don't work!" For individuals who find it difficult to follow a diet,or who are not successful with dieting there are alternatives. Individuals who are obese chronic dieting may not be the answer. We know that there are various reasons that contribute to the state of obesity. Medical conditions, related to one's body's regulation of weight, mixed with emotional factors are often too much for someone to overcome. Once the human body stores an excess amount of fat (the most obese people accumulate over 50% of their body mass as fat), one's health rapidly spirals downward unless aggressive steps are taken to combat the obesity condition.

Fortunately, successful long-term weight loss and weight maintenance can be achieved for individuals with a genotype that causes them to become severely obese. Bariatric surgeons have refined procedures over the years and even developed new methods (such as laparoscopic surgery) to combat obesity (refer to chapter 10). Healthy Conscious Eating does not rule out surgical intervention to obesity when surgery is appropriate and less invasive methods have failed; but surgical intervention for obesity should be a last resort. Even with the help of a surgical procedure, one still has to make choices and use Healthy Conscious Eating strategies. Remember, the goal of Healthy Conscious Eating from a psychological, and social standpoint is to know yourself and to integrate habits which defeat an unhealthy eating regimen. When you have established an unhealthy eating regimen your body has adapted to your abits by expressing protection allowing you to gain unhealthy amounts of fat leading to poor health and adverse metabolic consequences. When the human body has spent over 2 million years evolving to the point where it can store fat to survive the winter famine, there will be some people whose gene pool allow them to be too successful at storing fat and who will need medical intervention to survive in this new millenium when food is too available for this genotype.

Whether you atempt surgical intervention for weight loss or nonsurgical means Healthy Conscious Eating plays a "key role." Healthy Conscious Eating helps create self-awareness about your unhealthy eatingregimen, and helps you develop a plan that will work. Healthy Conscious Eating can help to create a more compassionate and forgiving attitude toward your goals. Rigid thinking (like perfect adherance to a restrictive diet) can cause feelings of guilt when strayed from. Gradually, replace the mechanisms that maintain an unhealthy eating regimen with self-exploration and acceptance, knowledge and education, social and psychological support.

Finally, we want everyone to be aware that when you consciously decrease the amount of food you are eating with surgical intervention or without, BE AWARE    that you are at a high risk for becoming depressed. Denial of any enjoyed activity; eating, sex, exercise, recreation, even work is a major cause of depression. Dieting and depression are "D" words linked in history back to the beginning of the end of cavemen and company. As soon as your food intake goes below your body's usual level you change serotonin levels in your brain which can cause depression. If you are already having depressed moods, it would be wise to see a psychotherapist and consider starting medication to treat depression before you try to change your diet or consider a surgical intervention.

Other unusual things can happen to you while you are losing weight. All of us resist change even to those points of our life we dislike (although it is easier to adjust to our improvement in life than a change for the worse). It is not unusual to feel upset as you lose weight because your body begins to change visually—even if this is what you want. I can be especially upsetting if you have children and they do not recognize you. If a small child thinks of his mom or dad as the biggest person in the room and then bypasses you for a heavier person it will initially upset both of you (but usually not for long). Again, a change as radical as a change in appearance an set off reactions in the subconscious and unconscious parts of the psyche that cause powerful, often unwanted emotions to surface. If you become aware of uncomfortable feelings while trying to change your habits, dietary or otherwise, seek professional help from a psychotherapist. A book like this is often only the beginning of a journey of self discovery.

Healthy Conscious Eating is not a cure-all for all food related problems. This book can be a useful tool that can assist you in developing insight so you can take appropriate steps to change your unhealthy eating regimen!

# Chapter 9
## Developing a Behavioral Modification Plan for Weight Loss

Let's Talk! With everything that's going on in your life, you have to sit back occasionally and wonder, "What is really important to me?" The answer is obvious, or it should be obvious to most, it is your health and your family's health. Take the time to create a healthy environment for you and your family by incorporating healthy conscious eating, and increased activity levels. Create the time to improve your health. Ask yourself, "How much does weight affect my quality of life?" Make it a priority to find time to foster better communication and health for you and your family. (Time is the one thing that you cannot speed up or slow down nor can you ever have enough of). Time can never be recaptured once it is lost. So unless time is managed effectively to meet your needs and obligations, nothing that you do can be managed effectively either.

The first step in managing your time effectively is to determine where does all your time go. Once that is determined, you can begin to implement healthy, positive changes accordingly. Most people when they create a plan realize that they have more discretionary time than once thought. When devising your behavioral modification plan, do it for the right reasons. External reasons can help you begin these changes and possibly lose weight, but any weight lost for external reasons are rarely permanent. People who keep weight off lose it for themselves because they are aware of the adverse health consequences that accompany obesity and they are committed to losing the excess weight and keeping it off. People who lose weight for superficial reasons usually regain their weight. When weight loss is permanent, it occurs because of lifestyle changes and the individual sticking with those changes for life. Make changes that you can live with, changes that are minimal and non-threatening. If you cannot envision yourself staying with those changes, do not even consider them. Do not fool yourself, disregard those changes and incorporate others.

Changes to consider can be as subtle as ordering and eating a hamburger and a small order of french fries as opposed to a cheeseburger and a super-sized order of french fried potatoes that is commonly advertised as a price saving combo meal. You can switch from ice cream to frozen fruits or yogurts. If you are opposed to jogging, you can walk in the park or shopping mall. You can park you vehicle further away from the supermarket when grocery shopping and further away from your office building door at work. Utilize the stairs at work more than you are currently doing now. And if you truly enjoy and must have high calorie desserts after a meal at home, maybe after dinner you can take a walk, return and then have the dessert. These changes may seem minor and insignificant but they are not. It is the small inconsequential changes mentioned that you can gradually incorporate into your present lifestyle that develops into permanent change.

It is not wise to diet by starvation or extreme dieting. When you diet, you in essence limit two vital components of nourishment (energy)—carbohydrates and total calories. The result is a short-term weight loss of maybe a few pounds over a relatively short period of time and then a rapid weight gain once you return to your old eating habits. Diets that limit caloric intake to less than 1,000 calories a day fools your body into thinking that it is starving. Your body will react to this perceived famine by lowering its basal metabolic rate. Your basal metabolic rate slows, your weight will reduce slowly. When you re-introduce food back into your lifestyle and normal consumption resumes, your fat cells and glycogen storage will quickly refill. Your basal metabolic rate will remain lowered for a while thereafter, and continue to burn calories slowly and you have the possiblity of gaining your weight back quickly plus additional weight due to your slower metabolic rate.

It is important to choose a healthy conscious eating strategy that you can successfully incorporate into your present lifestyle. The plan should include learning different stress management skills to effectively deal with everyday stressors. The plan should be strategic to incorporate interventions for night time eating, inappropriate snacking and improper food selections or other behaviors identified from your food diary. The plan should also allow you to learn how to select and prepare healthy foods and to incorporate increased activity levels. Learning to eat healthy and having the ability to manage stress effectively coupled with increased activity levels can lead to permanent weight loss and a healthier, happier lifestyle.

A healthier lifestyle is important as you grow older. As you age your total energy expenditure decreases as well as your muscular energy utilization. Simply stated, because of less muscle mass you use less energy. At age 30 it is estimated that non-muscle energy (vital organs, brain, etc.,) consumption is between 30%-40% of your total energy usage but by age 70, it is estimated that your non-muscle utilization of energy increases to approximately 50%. This change in usage of calories mandates that you incorporate good nutrition into your lifestyle and increase activity levels to avoid weight gain as you age.

Let's Talk! Anyone who is more than 20 percent over their ideal body weight for their age, sex, and height should discuss weight loss and increased activity levels with a physician. Sudden weight changes may cause extreme fatigue and exhaustion. Fad and/or very restricted diets can be dangerous and may lead to vitamin deficiency diseases. A gradual reduction in the amount of food eaten can result in a weight loss of 2 or

3 pounds a week, an overall loss of 10 pounds a month. Increased activity levels are value because it increases your body's metabolic rate and gives you a sense of well-being and relative freedom from fatigue. Strength training activities will increase the proportion of weight loss from body fat and will help protect your muscles.

It is now time to step back and take inventory of your lifestyle and where the bulk of your time is devoted. How much of your time do you spend either sleeping, lounging or sitting behind a desk at work. If you find that you are inactive the majority of your leisure time maybe it is time to re-adjust your lifestyle. Instead of spending evenings and weekends in front of the television, you could take a walk or bike ride. Instead of talking to a friend or love one who happens to call you on the telephone, ask that person to meet you at a nearby safe park or shopping mall for a walk and talk session. With proper planning you can gradually incorporate new behavioral changes into your lifestyle.

When doing so, remember to allow for flexibility and attempt only one or two changes at a time. You should view your weight loss attempt as a systematic process. A process that is detailed and implemented with a step by step plan for action to achieve the results you desire. Understand and process the information you have learned from this guide. Calculate your present resting metabolic rate, your new resting metabolic rate for weight loss, your current BMI and set your short term goals. Become aware of your relationship with food and focus on change. Understand the problem and focus on behaviors to implement change. Act in a concrete consistent manner. Institute positive rewards for achieving your goals and staying focus. Modify your behavior to increase or reinforce new behaviors. Utilize your energy and efforts to create a positive energy flow and environment. Use active behavioral strategies to integrate change into your daily life that reflects a healthy lifestyle and pretty soon you begin to sense that you are becoming more of the kind of person you want to be. When incorporating change into your present lifestyle remember to include the steps of behavioral change which are:

1) Medical Clearance.
2) Knowledge & Understanding of Nutrition.
3) Understanding and Managing Stress effectively.
4) Increrased activity levels that agree with your lifestyle and time.

## Medical Clearance:

Before you undertake a weight loss program, you should consult with your physician. (Even though primary care physicians are not advising their obese and overweight patients to lose weight despite our federal government guidelines, Healthy People 2000 & 2010 that recommend they do). Despite their reluctancce it is always advisable to consult with a health care professional to ensure that a medical disorder has not caused your weight problem. You should request a complete and thorough physical examination prior to undertaking any increasd level of exertion regimen, especially if you have been sedentary for quite a while.

## Health and Nutrition:

Reducing dietary fat alone without reducing calories will not promote weight loss. You will need to reduce overall calories. Knowing what to eat doesn't always mean that you will always choose to eat healthy. It is important to choose a healthy eating plan that you can successfully incorporate into your lifestyle. The plan should incorporate learning the necessary skills to effectively deal with stress. The plan should incorporate learning the necessary skills to effectively deal with stress; to eliminate or reduce night time eating and it should also teach you how to select and prepare healthy foods.

Most people experience pleasure in a variety of settings and it is important to realize change will not come easy. There is no one way to achieve weight loss and there is no right or wrong way; you must follow guidelines that wrok for you as an individual. Your initial goal should be to reduce your body weight by 10% over six months. This amount can usually reduce related risk factors. Learning to eat healthy and having the ability to deal with stress effectively coupled with increased activity levels can lead to permanent weight loss and a healthier lifestyle. A healthier lifestyle is important as you grow older. The dibursement and utilization of energy as you age changes dramatically.

Good keys to choosing a healthy meal is to choose meals low in fat (saturated fat and cholesterol). Choose meals that include plenty of grains, fruits, and vegetables. Plan meals that contain a variety of foods and are low in sugar. If you consume alcohol, do so in moderation. Listen to your internal cues for hunger such as fatigue, weakness,

decreased concentration, headaches or hunger pangs. Hunger pangs are pains in your abdominal region which occur in the early stages of hunger or fasting and are correlated with contractions of the empty stomach of intestines—(Merriam Webster's Medical Dictionary 1995 edition…) Hunger pangs should not always be interpreted as an indication of hunger during weight loss. The feeling of hunger is a complex physiological experience.

True hunger is triggered by the nutritional needs of your body and the feeling of emptiness in your stomach. Hunger can indicate several things. You are probably feeling these pangs because your stomach has been stretched due to overweight and it will continue to produce the hunger pangs for larger amounts of foods until its size is reduced. Reduction in stomach size can occur over a period of time.

### Managing Stress Effectively:

Perhaps the best approach to stress management is a general diverse approach. No single method is uniformly successful. Stress can have varying affects on your body weight. Stress can cause a weight gain due to cravings for salt, fat and sugars to counteract tension caused by stress.

Stress can be an underlying factor for overeating. Re-enforce or attain other coping skills for stress that will allow you to manage the urge to eat under stressful situations. Use behavioral skills you have learned (relaxation and positive self-talk), to relax and to stay in control.

### Behavior Modification:

Utilize new life strategies to incorporate new positive behaviors to enhance your control over your eating. Reduce nightime eating and high fat snacking. Understand the physiological, nutritional and psychological aspects of weight gain and weight loss. Behaviors are learned both good ones and bad ones. Set short-term goals to measure your success and build motivation. If you find yourself weakening re-adjust your goals to help regain motivation.

### Increasing Activity Levels:

The goals of increased activity levels are to improve oxygen delivery and metabolic processes, build strength and endurance, decrease body fat, and improve movement in muscles and joints. Incorporate aerobic and other physical activities into your lifestyle for healthy living. Utilize your newfound time and vigor to maintain motivation to increase your activity levels. It is best to incorporate both cardiorespiratory endurance as well as resistance training when embarking on a fitness program for weight loss. The key to attaining and maintaining increased activity levels is to find activities that are exciting, challenging and satisfying to you. If you have never weight trained before, you can and will be amazed at how quickly your body will adapt to your new activities.

The physiological adaptations to these different types of activities are different. Yet both have proven effective in improving physical capacity and health. Endurance activities improves the efficiency and functions of your cardiorespiratory system, thus allowing your body to function more efficiently and to burn fat quicker due to increased enzyme action and oxidation of glycogen. Endurance training should be something you enjoy because of the amount of time you need to actively involve yourself in those activities when pursuing weight loss.

Resistance training helps to make improvements to your skeletal muscle and increase your lean muscle mass. Resistance training can increase your resting metabolic rate. Resistance training should consist of 8-10 different activities performed at least twice weekly for a minimum of 3 sets and 8-10 repetitions. Choose the correct weight when starting out and progress at your pace. Select a weight that you can lift 10 to 15 times while maintaining good form. When you advance to a stage where it is relatively easy lifting the weight you initially selected, it is time to advance to a heavier weight. Breathe properly when weight lifting by inhaling as you lower the weights and exhaling as you lift the weight. Go slowly, each repetition should use precise movement for muscular enhancement and take several seconds to complete. Protect your back at all times, when squatting and lift with your legs rather than leaning forward and jerking with your back.

Physical fitness results from adaptation to progressive overload.

Progressive overload simply means asking your body to do a little bit more than what it is accustomed to doing. Your body adapts in ways specific to the overload you place upon it. Adaptations occur in your energy production systems, the structure and function of your cardiorespiratory system, your blood chemistry, your bone and joint strength and in other systems as well. When you increase your cardiorespiratory activity levels, your aerobic system that produce energy for long-term muscular work will get better at producing energy thus allowing even more activities. A structured plan that encompasses both muscular strength training and cardiorespiratory endurance can improve your muscle tone and produce a leaner more efficient body.

If you want to lose weight, you'll have to eat fewer calories than you expend. You can do this either by cutting your caloric intake or by increasing your activity level. A combination of both with an emphasis on incresing your activity is the best choice. When cutting down on calories, aim for the amount needed daily to maintain your goal weight, basal metabolic rate and current energy level; not your present weight. Keep in mind, however, that your body is smart and will strive to maintain its current levels of fat storage for survival. If you deprive your body of necessary calories, your body will think that you are starving and it will do its very best to keep you from dying of hunger. The only way to counteract this perceived starvation is to lower your caloric intake gradually while increasing your caloric expenditure. Drastically cutting back on food alone will cause your body to burn calories at a slower rate.

Increased activity levels and healthy conscious eating will keep your body burning fat instead of muscles. Don't underestimate the importance of setting realistic goals. Research has found that your body wants to maintain its heavy weight. When you create a drastic deficit in fat storage your body will respond out of survival. So do not set goals that are counter productive to your weight loss attempt. Try losing 10% of your baseline weight and keeping it off for about 6 months and then aim for another 10% reduction in body fat.

# Chapter 10
## Surgical Interventions for Weight Loss

Let's Talk! Obesity is a major health problem a serious, chronic disease that has reached epidemic porportions in large part because our government and business communities view surgical intervention to obesity is a cosmetic option rather than a medical intervention. Understanding the health risk of severe obesity, it's definition, assessment, prevention and interventions can allow you to better combat this disease. Having biological family members with severe obesity increases your risk and the risk of your children developing obesity. The magnitude of risk increases with the severity of obesity that develops in each family member. You should understand that weight gain in adulthood can be harmful to your health and should not be considered the normal part of aging. Understanding the health risk associated with weight gain and attempting to prevent it before it reaches the state of severe obesity is the best strategy. Knowing and monitoring your weight (BMI) is important in weight management. BMI correlates significantly with total body fat. It is important to know your BMI.

| | |
|---|---|
| Table 1 | |
| Healthy Weight | |
| **Weight** | **BMI** |
| Healthy Weight | 18.6—24.9 |
| Overweight | 25.0—29.9 |
| Obese | 30.0—39.9 |
| Morbid obese (severe) | > 40.0 |

Long-term weight loss programs designed to obtain a healthy weight for individuals whose BMI is equal to or greater than 40, often requires surgery. Physicians have developed surgical procedures that limit food consumption or absorption in order to facilitate weight loss. Among these surgical procedures are 1) restrictive procedures which include the Roux-en-Y Gastric Bypass, and Adjustable and Non-Adjustable Gastric Banding Procedures, and various forms of gastroplasties such as the vertical banded gastroplasty, and 2) mixed restrictive and malabsorptive procedures such as Biliopancreatic Bypass. These procedures can be performed as an open procedure using a 12" abdominal incision or can be performed in some instances using a minimally invasive laparoscopic surgical technique where four to six 1/2–2" incisions are used to place tubes (trochars) which can be used to do "video surgery." The laparoscopic technique utilizes a camera to assist the surgeon performing the operation and the surgical instruments are passed through the trochars while the surgeons view a video screen to help them operate, similar to playing video poker. Convalescence time may be reduced and post-operative pain may also be reduced allowing you to return to work or to your normal activities quicker because the abdominal muscles are not cut and pried open with metal retractors so that the surgeons can get their four hands into the abdomen to manually handle the body's organs and tissue (See illustrations 1 & 2).

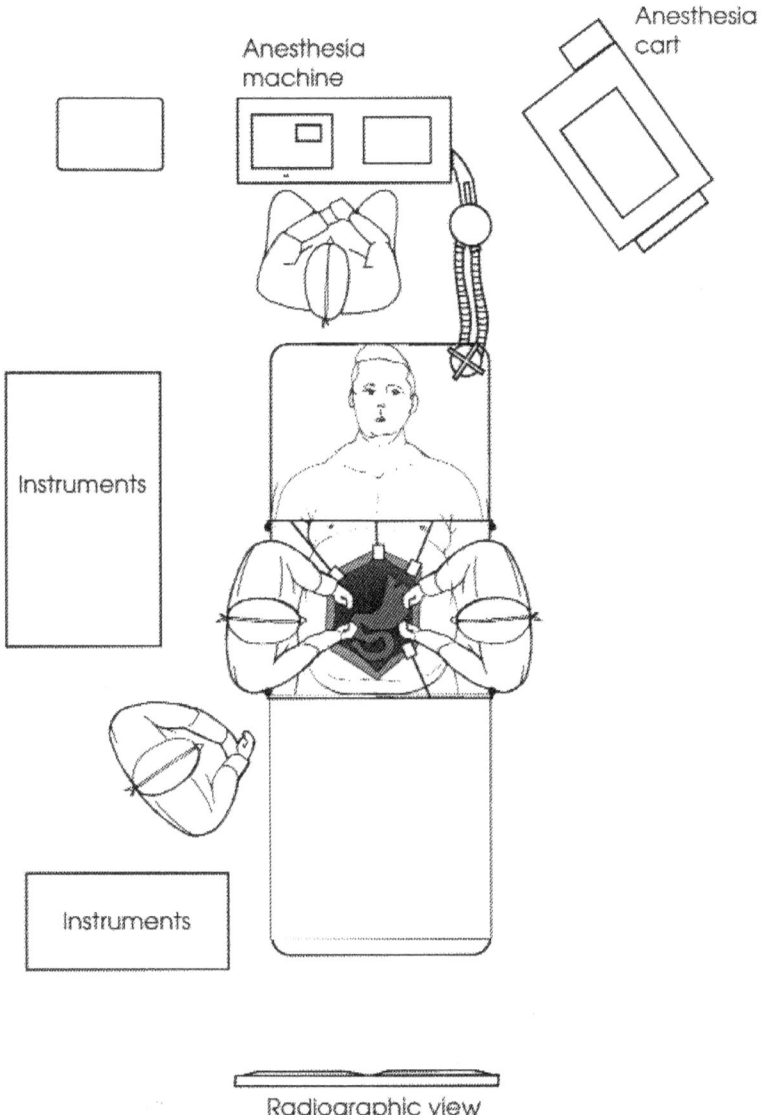

*Illustration # 1, traditional operating room technique where surgeon and assistant place their instruments and hands through the stretched open incision made in the abdomen so that they view the tissues directly.*

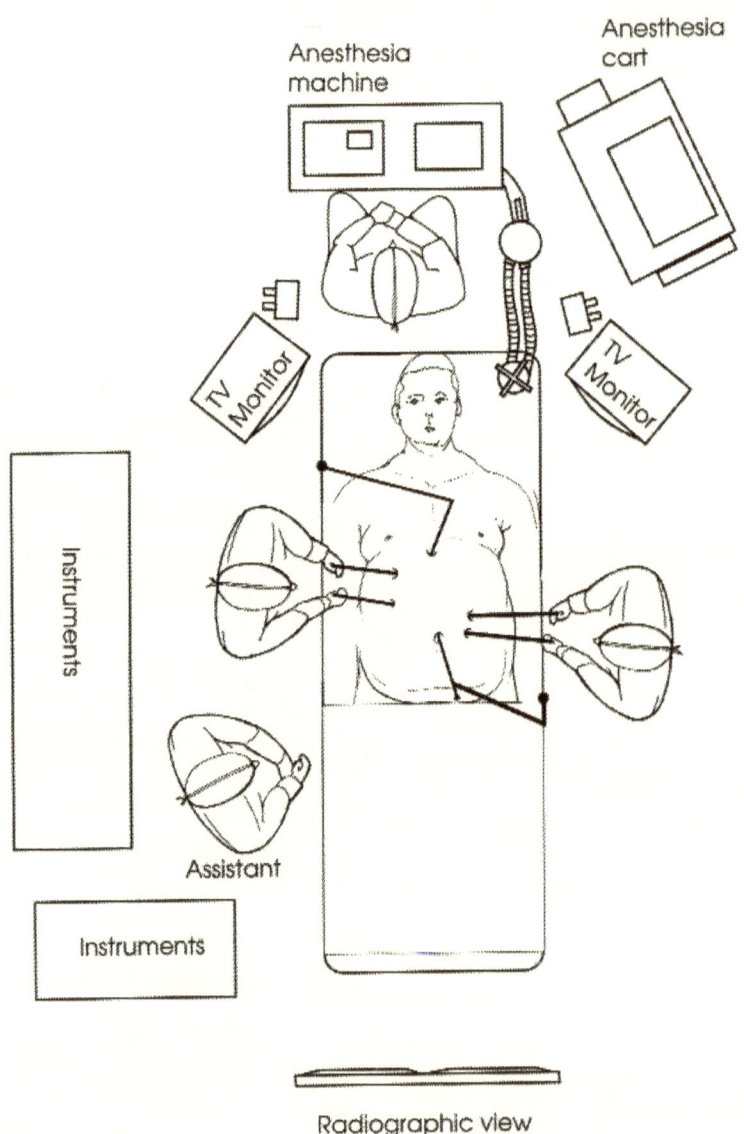

Radiographic view

*Illustration # 2, Laparoscopic set-up with surgeon and assistant using instruments inserted thru trochars and viewing surgery on video screen where camera is moved by a computerized mechanical arm under the voice control of the primary surgeon.*

This chapter is written as a resource of information for those individuals who have decided to utilize surgical intervention as a means to combat obesity and to achieve and maintain a healthy weight. This chapter will describe the stages of obesity, and its causes and effects; and describe the major surgical procedures to combat obesity.

The National Institutes of Health (NIH) estimates that at least 1.5 million people in the United States is morbidly obese. People who suffer from morbid obesity (BMI > 40) are suffering from a physical illness and are at an increased risk of developing numerous other illnesses. By definition, you are considered morbidly obese when your BMI reaches 40 or above (See table # 1). Many physicians feel if your BMI is 35 or more and you have an accompanying illness related to the obesity such as diabetes or hypertension, then you too are morbidly obese. At this point of obesity, the excess weight is so great that it becomes potentially life threatening. A morbidly obese adult has only one-third the chance of living to age 65 as that of a person who is of normal weight. Insurance companies will often not insure people whose weight is 30% above normal because their rate of heart disease is 50%—70% times higher than people of normal weights (yet, they talk out of the other side of their mouth when surgical therapy is requested, by denying how lifesaving such therapy can be). Surgical intervention to treat obesity must be part of a serious long-term commitment to your health. Surgery is and should be a last resort; not only do you need to be sure that surgery is the right choice for you but you should have failed at less invasive attempts at weight loss.

If surgery is the appropriate choice for you, then you should enter this commitment understanding that you must change your lifestyle. You must make a commitment to change your lifestyle and focus on your health. Several medical[1], and nutritional[2] organizations, as well as the National Institutes of Health (NIH)[3], have adopted guidelines to help physicians determine which of their patients should be referred for surgical intervention for obesity. Individuals who meet these guidelines and criterias would be candidates for surgical treatment based on medical studies that have examined the risk and benefit of those procedures. Insurance companies, however, do not always allow their clients to have this type of procedure even though they pay over $3,000 per year to obtain medial benefits coverage. Insurance companies have often excluded all obesity treatments from their contracts using the excuse that some treatments are not effective. Although most states allow an insurance company to exclude any treatment they want to, ethical insurance companies have rarely excluded life saving treatments. The exclusion of a life threatening condition treatments demonstrates why health companies need to be overseen by government agencies. Left to their own devices, some insurance companies discriminate against any disease to maximize profits.

Table 2

## *DETERMINATION OF OBESITY BY BMI

| CLASSIFICATION | BMI |
| --- | --- |
| Overweight | 25—29 |
| Obesity Class I | 30—34 |
| Obesity Class II | 35—39 |
| Obesity Class III | >40 |

*Table taken from Healthy People 2010, American Obesity Association; 1250 24th St. NW, Suite 300 · Washington, DC 20037· Tel: (202) 776-7711· Fax: (202) 776-7712

In general, surgical procedures performed to achieve weight loss for morbid obesity are divided into two surgical categories,
1) malabsorptive and 2)restrictive. Malabsorptive procedures decrease intestinal absorption of food by the individual and restrictive procedures decrease the amount of food you are able to ingest. Some surgical procedures combine the two mechanisms so that they are both restrictive and malabsorptive.

1. World Health Organization.http://www.who.int/htm.
2. Shape Up America! Foundation.http://www.shapeup.org/htm.
3. National Institutes of Health.http://www.nih.gov/htm.

Roux-en-Y Gastric Bypass

(The Gold Standard)Let's Talk! To qualify as a candidate you must be at least one hundred pounds over your ideal body weight or have a BMI equal to, or above 40. There are circumstances whereas your BMI can be lower. For instance, if your excess weight is accompanied with serious medical problems that may be lessened or greatly improved with significant weight loss. Usually documentation of historically failing less invasive options for weight loss such as diets and/or medication is necessary. Individuals opting for surgical interventions are advised to carefully consider their selection of a surgical procedure. Before choosing a surgical procedure you should explore the advantages and disadvantages of each procedure. Look at what obesity surgery program is suitable for you, based on your medical history, present conditions and expectations of the outcome of the surgical procedure. A weight management/obesity treatment center program should be equipped with health professionals who are well informed and can create individual treatment plans to keep you focused and on track. The staff should consist of physician(s), dietitian(s), nurse(s), exercise physiologist(s), social worker/behaviorist(s), psychologist(s),and bariatric surgeon(s) where surgical intervention for obesity is offered.

The program should offer steps to help you control your weight; which are within your reach through behavior modification, healthy conscious eating, increased activity levels, and possibly medication. The program should offer flexible treatment options that can be modified for individual needs. The staff should be able to provide different types of weight control options using individual and group support to address the psychological aspects of weight gain/loss, pre-operative education, assessments, and post-operative follow-up care.

Some treatment facilities provide a comprehensive treatment plan that includes a multidisciplinary approach utilizing nutritional, physiological, and psychological testing assessments and regular perioperative interactions with staff members. This is done to better assess the necessary lifestyle changes that will become a part of the new you. After gastric bypass surgery, you should anticipate regular appointments with the surgeon. This is necessary to follow and monitor your progress and to ensure you are on your way to improved health.

Gastric Bypass is both a restrictive and malabsorptive surgical procedure. The amount and types of food(s) you are able to ingest is restricted due to your reduced stomach capacity. The "new" reduced stomach capacity restricts your caloric consumption to only a few ounces of food at one time. The "new" smaller stomach (less than 2 ounces) is created by dividing your stomach into two compartments (a top compartment and a bottom compartment). This is usually done by placing at least four rows of staples between the two compartments using at least two staple gun cartridges for placing two rows of staples. The two staple guns are placed side by side and then the stomach is divided by cutting it between the two guns making a permanent scar that rarely comes undone or "breaks" even after prolonged time has elasped. With total separation, staple line failure is uncommon, but can still occur in the immediate post-operative period if post-operative directions are not followed.

The "new" small proximal stomach is then hooked to the rest of the bowel in a procedure originally described by a French surgeon named Roux which resembles a Y in its design (hence it is called "Roux's Y" or in French "Roux-en-Y"). The small bowel is divided approximately three feet from the end of the stomach. The lower end of the small intestine is joined to the upper half of the divided stomach by a small (1/2 inch in diameter) outlet. Now, when you consume calories (food), the food enters the top half of your "new stomach" and causes you to feel full due to the small capacity and the narrow new opening to the rest of the small intestine (the restricted outlet keeps the food from exiting the pouch prolonging the feeling of fullness). The food passes into the small intestine through the outlet (see illustration #3).

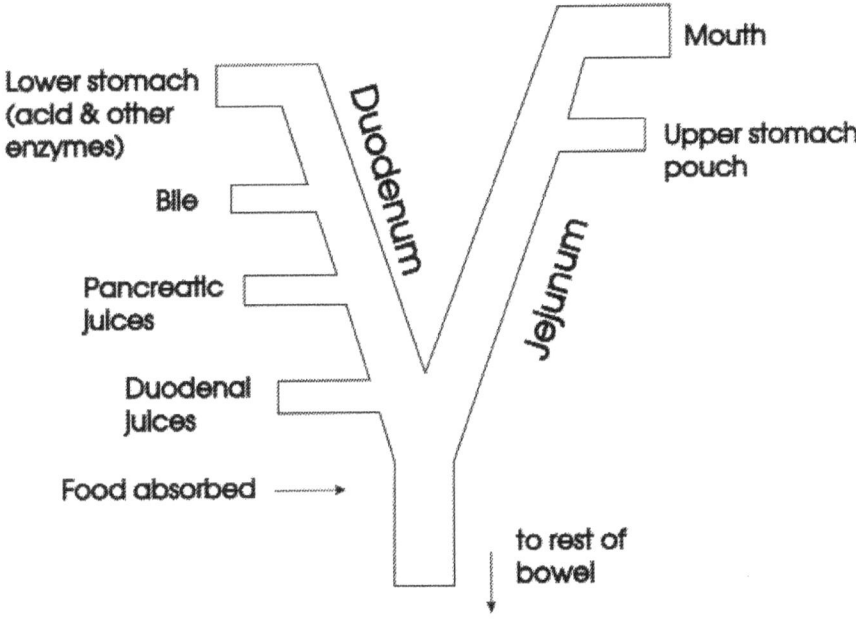

*Illustration # 3, The "new" small proximal stomach is hooked to the rest of the bowel. The small bowel is divided approximately three feet from the end of the stomach. The lower end of the small intestine is joined to the upper half of the divided stomach by a small outlet. Now, when you consume food, the food enters the top half of your "new" stomach and causes you to feel full due to the small capacity and narrow new opening to the rest of the intestine.*

In essence, you are getting the food to bypass the lower larger half of your stomach and the first three feet of the small intestine (thus decreasing the amount of food the small bowel absorbs, causing, malabsorption). Digestion still depends on the digestive juices from the lower half of the stomach, the duodenum and pancreas mixing with the food you consume through the smaller upper stomach pouch at the stem of the Y.

The gastric bypass surgery procedure does not alter or remove any other body organ and still allows for digestion, although, in a less effective manner. After surgery, **you will have to make changes to your lifestyle and eating habits.** You will usually be advised to remain on liquids for three weeks with a gradual progression to solids foods. You will need to chew food carefully to get a consistency that will slide through the new small gastric outlet channel or other intestinal connections without asking the recently traumatized bowel to work very hard until it has recovered from surgery. Since this procedure involves the re-routing of your small intestine so that food no longer passes through a portion of your stomach and small intestine during the digestive process, you have to chew your food much more completely. The food has to be chewed until it resembles toothpaste so it can pass through the small outlet leading to the small intestine. Also, acid, bile and enzymes that help dissolve proteins and help absorb fat no longer mix with the food until the two halves of the Y connect at the stem so that it is important to keep your food in your mouth chewing it long enough so that saliva can mix with it providing the enzymes the saliva secrete to help with the digestive process.

The gastric bypass also interrupts the digestive functions provided by the stomach in adding acid and other fluids to the food until the osmotic concentration of the mixture is maximized for absorption by the small intestine. The pylorus, the muscle at the distal end of the stomach, controls the exit of the food mixture to the rest of the intestine until the right **osmotic concentration** is obtained (the concentration or number of food particles per ounce of the food mixture). After the intestines are rearranged during gastric bypass, the new pouch has no way to control and monitor the osmotic concentration. If someone eats or drinks fluids with a high osmotic concentration such as ice cream, maple syrup or other concentrated "sweets" after a gastric bypass these fluids will cause small bowel irritation and produce a syndrome called **"dumping."** During the dumping syndrome, the small bowel is irritated causing the bowel to cramp producing diarrhea, abdominal pain with nausea and headache, flushing, and palpitations, and an overall feeling of malaise. These symptoms do not have to be experienced very often before one learns to avoid concentrated sweets or concentrated fats (another substance which often produces dumping).

Problems can develop during the first six months after the operation. You will need vitamin B12 supplements periodically, and routine office visits that include blood tests and a review of your nutritional status. The parts of the stomach and the small intestine, that are no longer in contact with food, (part 1 of the Y, illustration # 4), are the sites where vitamin B12, iron, and calcium are absorbed. Therefore it is imperative that you take a daily multi-vitamin and periodic injections of vitamin B12 after a gastric bypass since you cannot absorb these vitamins very effectively with the parts of the intestine that are in contact with the flow of food.

(See illustration # 4 below).

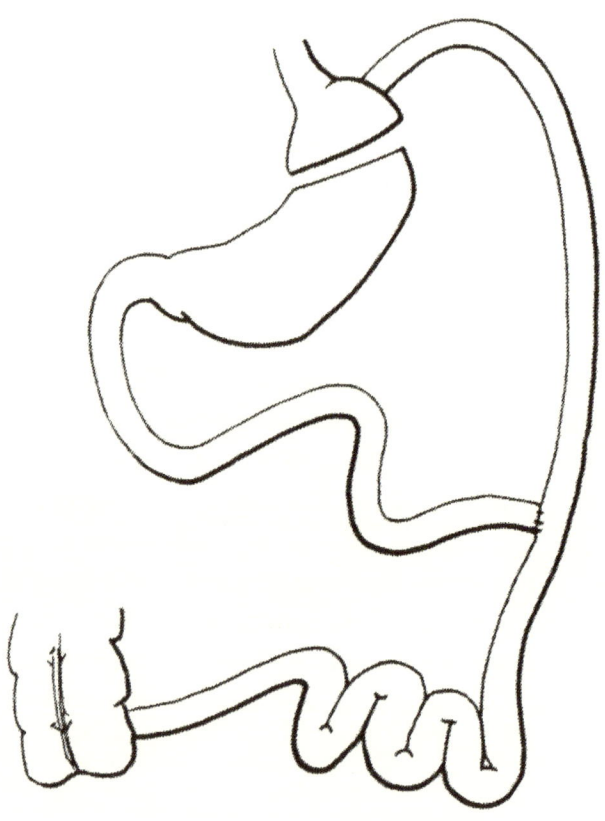

Other risks and problems associated with the gastric bypass procedure include the possible develop of pulmonary embolisms, hernia, gallstones, leakage from where the bowel is reconnected (the anastomoses), and/or infections. An infection caused by a leak at the anastomoses is one of the most serious complications that can occur after a gastric bypass. The surgeon makes sure during the operation that there are no leaks. However, the surgeon cannot move your body on the operating room table into all positions it needs to be flexed, like lacing your shoes, combing your hair or washing yourself. A leak occurs after a gastric bypass in less than 1 of 20 people who have surgery. These occur when one of the sutures or staples pull loose because the body is flexed or pulled in a way that pulls too much on the anastomosis causing a tear. Usually, when this happens, it needs to be fixed by a second operation, but occasionally it can heal without serious complications that can occur after a gastric bypass surgery. The hospital stay is usually 2 to 5 days, depending on recovery time and whether the procedure was performed laparoscopically or through the more traditional 10" midline incision.

At home convalescence after this usually is 2-5 weeks. You will be very tired for about two weeks after gastric bypass surgery resulting in extensive sleep while your body is healing its wound. During this time your stomach and intestines are healing from surgery hunger pangs are not unusual. It is not difficult to restrict food intake initially to one or two ounces of soft food or four to eight ounces of a high protein, low calorie liquid diet such as Slim-Fast, Sugar-Free Carnation-Instant Breakfast, Smoothie King products, or other similar products four to six times a day. You should start eating from smaller plates, such as a coffee saucer or a soup bowl.

Walking should be used as your major activity to help increase blood flow to enhance healing and to stimulate the release of stored fat so that weight can be lost while caloric intake is decreased. **You do not get better sitting on a couch watching daytime soap operas.** It is better to walk 15-30 minutes 2 to 6 times a day and nap between periods of activity and food consumption.

**Restrictive Operations Including:**   Gastric Bands
Adjustable Gastric Bands
Vertical Banded Gastroplasties


Restricting the amount of food that someone can eat at a meal is an obvious means of inducing weight loss. Ever since surgeons began treating gastric and peptic ulcer diseases at the end of the 19th century, operations which include restriction (removal) of part of the stomach have produced both short-term and long-term weight loss. In the 1970's, surgeons began using this information, which was over half a century old, to design operations for obesity. The initial designs all involved alterations to the stomach, technically called **"gastroplasty"** in medical terms, where the volume of the stomach was reduced. Over the last 30 years, we have learned that these procedures can produce weight loss, but the conditions that must be met for this to occur are very stringent or restrictive (safety, health, insurance, surgical appropriateness).

The normal unaltered stomach can hold 1 to 1.5 liters of fluid or food. In morbidly obese people, the stomach must be reduced to under 2 ounces or 30 milliliters for a significant amount of weight loss (50 pounds or more). Furthermore, the opening of the exit outlet out of this pouch must be less than 12mm, or ½inch in diameter. Historically, this degree of restriction in size of the pouch and outlet diameter has been hard to achieve in the stomach because it is pliable and active with its muscular contractions. The only way to maintain the exit outlet size has been to wrap a nondistensible device around the outlet, usually some form of plastic, silicone, or polypropelene material that will not stretch. The restriction of the size of the pouch can be created by dividing the stomach with staples, (Vertical Banded Gastroplasty), sutures, or bands made of these nondistensible plastics, silicones, or polypropelene materials. When a band is wrapped around the stomach that is made of one of these nondistensible substances to create both the pouch and the outlet restriction, the stomach does not have to be cut which decreases the risk of infection.

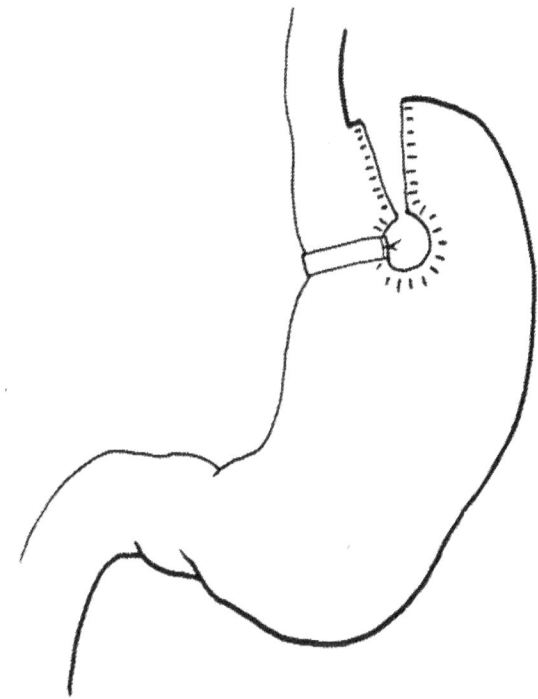

*Biliopancreatic bypass, this is a malabsorption procedure which shortens the length of the small intestine (bowel), where food can be absorbed by using approximately ½ the length of the bowel. This procedure can cause protein and vitamin deficiencies, especially of the fat soluble vitamins. It is an effective procedure and often is used when one of the other procedures proves ineffective.*

The most recent innovation made in banding procedure is to make the band adjustable by placing a ballon within the band used to create the pouch. The outlet restriction can then be adjusted fine tuning the restriction so that it will be tight enough. The band is made adjustable by connecting the ballon within the structure of the band to an "access port" which is left embedded in the abdominal muscles by a connecting link of tubing.

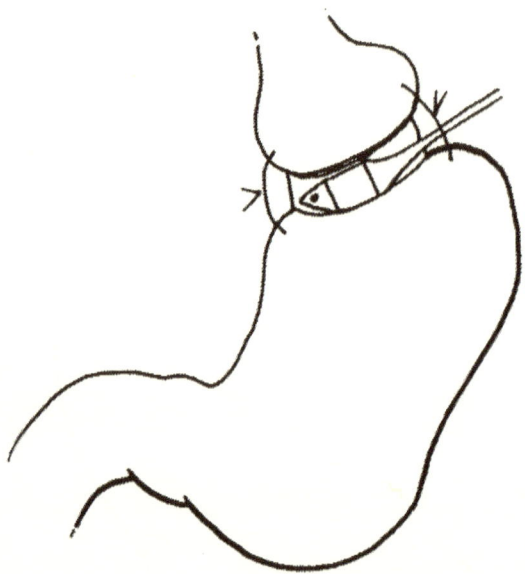

Once recovery from the operation is complete (so that the swelling associated with the surgical trauma has resolved), fluid maybe added to the ballon to tighten the outlet restriction by accessing the access port with the help of a radiologist.

The adjustment are done by radiologists. The radiologist is able to guide a needle attached to a fluid filled syringe to the access port using a fluroscopic x-ray machine. Fluid is added, the tightness of the outlet restriction is judged by watching radiolucent fluid, such as barium, and then the needle and syringe are withdrawn. These devices are called adjustable gastric bands and there are two companies making these devices, BioEnterics Corporation, CA., and Obtech Corporation of—Switzerland. Only the BioEnterics brand is currently available in the United States.

Adjustable gastric bands have become a popular type of obesity treatment in Europe, Australia, Central and Southern America because the bands have been designed to be placed using minimally invasive surgical techniques. Surgeons use a video camera, the laporoscope, and 5-6 small

1/4—2" incisions rather than an 8"–12" abdominal incision. Over 40,000 of these devices have been placed worldwide to treat obesity from September 1993 to June 2000. In the United States, the placement of This device to treat obesity has been investigated by a trial monitor of the Federal Food and Drug Administration (FDA), that started in 1995. The company, BioEnterics Corporation, was scheduled to seek approval to market this device by presenting the results of their trial in June of 2000 to the FDA. The status of the devise (approved for marketing, rejected as unsafe, or not resolved pending further data collection), should be available by December of 2001, this information is available by contacting the FDA, http://www.fda.gov/ora/compliance/html), or by contacting the BioEnterics Corporation at 1-805-684-3045, or through their website at (http://www.bioenterics.com/us/contact/index.html).

The BioEnterics company will have to train surgeons to place the device even if it is approved this year. Do not expect this device to be available in your town or location until sometimes in the year 2001.

Biliopancreatic Bypass (BPB) or
Duodenal Switch Procedure (DSP):

The other major type of obesity procedure available in this country to treat obesity is a major malabsorption procedure which shortens the length of the small intestine (bowel), where food can be absorbed by using approximately ½ the length of the bowel. This procedure can cause protein and vitamin deficiencies, especially of the fat soluble vitamins so that many surgeons, this author included, do not recommend this operation as a primary weight loss treatment. It is an effective procedure, however, and often is used when one of the other procedures, proves ineffective.

Both the biliopancreatic bypass (BPB) and the duodenal switch procedure (DSP) have been used before 1980 in the United States and the BPB before that in Europe and Canada. Both differ from early versions of malabsorptive procedures classified as "small bowel bypasses" or "jejunoileal bypasses" by having bacteriostatic body fluids flow through the part of the bowel excluded from the flow of food. These design differences prevent the accumulation of bacteria (germs) in the bypass bowel. This can lead to the absorption of toxic bacteria side products, causing acute organ failure and/or cirrhosis and other inflammatory problems including joint pains.

Both procedures reduce the size of the stomach, less food is consumed at each meal than usual. The procedures are not usually considered restrictive, however, because they allow more intake than the ½ cup of food allowed after gastric bypass or gastroplasty.

This has made some people question why most American, European and Australian surgeons recommend gastric bypass or gastric banding procedures rather than the BPB or DSP. The primary reason it is not recommended is because of the number of people who develop malnutrition or vitamin deficiencies after BPB and DSP. It is usually possible to prevent protein and vitamin deficiencies if an individual closely monitors protein intake and takes large quantities of supplemental vitamins. It is a minority of people who find it too difficult to follow this rigid protocol that get into trouble. The seriousness of the problems which can develop when a patient resists regular medical follow-up and the intake of supplements, however, prevents many surgeons from offering this to people initially because there is no reliable way to make these procedures successful.

The BPB, and DSP, also produce major weight loss by malabsorption of Food. This means that people who have these procedures experience diarrhea for the rest of their lives. This can be socially inhibiting and interfere with job performance. We worry that the people who are attracted to these procedures maybe are looking for a way to continue an unhealthy eating syndrome, which exhibits a denial of the process that got them into trouble in the first place.

Even though we have stated the unfavorable aspects of these procedures, if you weigh over 400 pounds or have a BMI over 65 (kg/m^2), you should evaluate these procedures as one of your options because you have already proven that you are very effective at absorbing food. Most surgeons will be open to discussing a wide range of options with you and other obese people. Even if you weigh over 500 pounds, you have at least a 2%-5% chance of having trouble absorbing enough protein to keep your muscle mass and albumin levels at healthy levels. We recently had to revise a BPB procedure. Revisions usually requires a procedure to lengthen the amount of small bowel in contact with the flow of food in a patient who was consuming 120 grams of protein a day (twice the amount of protein people need to consume normally to stay healthy or stay healthy after a gastric bypass or gastric banding procedure). The patient was an individual who charted their food intake and was amazed that someone could physically consume enough protein to stay healthy after a BPB procedure. This case was unusual (less than 1 in 20). The patient was very dissatisfied that the surgeon who performed the procedure stated that a BPB was the only procedure that could help the patient lose the extra weight. (The patient felt the surgeon oversold the BPB procedure).

### Risks Associated with Surgery:

In defense of the surgeon, people who develop complications rarely feel that their surgeon gave them the right amount of information preoperatively; these procedures have at least a 1% mortality (death rate), a 3%-8% serious complication rate (requiring another operation or a prolonged hospital stay depending on the burden of co-morbid medical problems one has), and a 10%-30% minor complication rate (including all events which led to additional discomfort or expense).

JUST REMEMBER that **morbid** obesity, the **disease** one has to have to qualify for all these surgical procedures, is a disease that leads most people to die at a much younger age than other Americans and leads to the development or worsening of a long list of associated serious medical conditions including diabetes, heart disease, breathing problem, strokes, cancers, high blood pressure, leg swelling, stress incontinence, arthritis (especially low back pain, hip pain and knee pain), sleep apnea, gallstones, elevated cholesterol and triglyceride levels, depression, menstrual irregularities infertility, and social problems. Social problems includes loss of employment, or early retirement due to disability, loss of employment, less chance of getting jobs you qualify for, less chance of completing your education, less chance of getting married, and a decreased quality of life.

Surgical treatment of obesity can produce sudden death, other major medical complications, or many minor inconvenience, but if you do not try to reducing your weight the life you live will not be as rich, nor as comfortable or fullfilling as your life would be if you lost 100, 200, 300 pounds or more. Most obese people deny how depressed they are by the constraints imposed on them by their obesity,(A MAJOR DISABILITY). Helen Keller, a blind and deaf young girl who overcame her disabilities at the turn of the century stated her philosophy—"Life is either an exciting adventure or nothing!" No one who choses to remain morbidly obese is looking at life as an exciting adventure. We choose to help people fight obesity through surgical therapy even though we suffer heartache with one of our patient's deaths, and/or the development of a serious complication. However, the joy we feel watching over 95% of our patients obtain a normal life after being inhibited by morbid obesity balances the few times a year one of our patients has a bad outcome. We do not minimize the risk each individual takes as they evaluate their options, understand, "You do not have a 1% chance of dying after an operation—You either live or die!" It is the quality of your life that you must consider, the needs of the people who are dependent on you, and whether you can obtain insurance to help damper the tradegy of your disability or death if you die prematurely because of your obesity or the associated disease burden, or die prematurely at the time of your operation while trying to improve your life and the lives of all those who depend on you. This is a monumental decision that only you can make. Only 1% of the morbidly obese people in America choose surgical therapy in any given year. Most people are too afraid of the risks associated with the operations that are currently offered, and are looking for less dangerous ways to treat obesity. Surgeons are trying to do less invasive procedures using laparoscopy—video surgery using multiply small incisions rather than one 6" –12" incision. New ideas; such as using a battery to stimulate the electrical activity of the stomach attempting to fool it and the brain into thinking that a large meal has just been consumed all the time, (an off shoot of the cardiac pacemaker technology), are in clinical trials. The National Institutes of Health asks scientist for proposals testing new ways of treating obesity and reserves money that can only be used if good ideas are identified.

Certain agencies within the federal government tell Congress and the media that obesity is now an epidemic. These agencies want everyone to know that obesity and its related diseases are the second most common cause of preventable death in America. They also recognize that cigarette/tobacco usage is decreasing, but that the number of children and adults who have become obese are increasing. We are killing ourselves by overeating. We need to stop this trend.

Let's Talk! We cannot help everybody **BUT,** we want to help you and your family. After reading this book, utilize the worksheets in the appendixes of this book. Develop a plan! Contact us! Plan for your future! Start by identifying your unhealthy eating syndrome actively trying to incorporate healthy conscious eating, and leading an active lifestyle! We can help you! BUT only you can take the first step! Our hands are reaching out to you! Walk toward us! Let us help! Each step you take with lesser burden, lightens your load, (give it to us), and improve your quality of life! We want to help you! We are here for you! Let's Talk! IMPROVE YOUR LIFE NOW!

# About the Authors

Louis Frank Martin, MD, FACS, FCCM, Bariatric Surgeon, Professor of Surgery, Louisiana State University Health Sciences Center in New Orleans, Dr. Martin is a nationally and internationally recognized general surgeon whose practice is dedicated to treating obesity. He has been involved in surgical treatments for obesity since 1983. He helped organize the first multi-disciplinary team to treat obesity at Penn State's College of Medicine in Hershey, PA. He moved to New Orleans in 1992, to become a professor of surgery and director of all adult weight loss services at LSUHSC. He has published numerous scientific and lay articles on the problems of obesity and has helped hundreds of obese individuals achieve & maintain a healthy weight. Dr. Martin has appeared on television and radio talk shows addressing obesity issues. He has been a member of the Executive Council of the American Society of Bariatric Surgeons 1996-1998.

Kenneth R. Bibbins, CEP., is an obesity specialist located in New Orleans, Louisiana. He has completed research and training in various areas of obesity treatments and clinical outcomes. He has been instrumental in developing clinical protocols pre-operatively and post-operatively for obese individuals pursuing surgical intervention to obesity. He now works as an exercise physiologist assisting clinically obese inviduals lose weight through healthy conscious eating, active lifestyles, and ridding themselves of an unhealthy eating syndrome through behavior modification, stress management and self awareness.

# *APPENDIX A*

Use this sheet to calculate your resting metabolic rate, BMI, your new caloric intake andyour fat percentage: Use this as a guide to measure your progress and success:

Name : _____Starting Date : _____

Age: ____Height ___(meters)Weight: ____(Kilograms) BMI: ____
Current Caloric intake: (RMR) _____daily calories presently consume
Actual calories you are consuming: _____ x 30=_____

Insert New Daily Calories: _____(1,200-1,300 Females;1,500 Males)
Insert actual calories here _____ — _____=_____
                (line 4)       (line 5)   (daily decrease)

Insert Daily Caloric Decrease: _____ x 7 days a week=_____wkly decrease Weekly Caloric decrease: _____/3,500 calories= _____possible wkly loss Insert Pounds from above line: _____this may be your weekly weight loss. Are you currently eating breakfast? Yes _____ No _____ Sometimes_____ How many times a day are you eating? _____ How many calories?____ List times of meals: 1ˢᵗ____ 2ⁿᵈ____ 3ʳᵈ____4ᵗʰ____5ᵗʰ_____ Any late night eating? Yes_____ No_____ if yes, why? Hunger_____ Habit_____ Current Coat/Jacket size: _____Current waist/belt size: _____ Current Blouse/shirt/neck size: _____Current slacks/pant size:_____

**Ideal Body Weight Calculations:** The below calculations suggest that a person's weight should be based on their height for optimal health:

Height: _____(meters) Weight:_____ (kilograms) Current BMI: _____ / 2.2= _____kilogram wgt. _____hgt.(inches) x 0.0254=_____ (wgt.in lbs.) (meters) _____x_____= _____ Desirable Body Mass: _____(BMI) (meters) (meters) (meters squared) Insert meters squared _____ x _____=_____ X 2.2=_____

(Desired BMI)

(ideal body weight)

## Desirable BMI by Age:

| AGE: | BMI: |
|------|------|
| 15-23 | 18-23 |
| 24-32 | 19-24 |
| | |
| 33-42 | 21-25 |
| 42—Over | 22-28 |

# APPENDIX B

**Calculations & Instructions:** The equation below use weight in kilograms.

**World Health Organization:** Calculations taken from the World Health Organization:Although not completely accurate can seve as a guide for calculating total **Energy Needs**.

Change weight/pounds to kilograms: Divide weight by 2.2: Example 200/2.2=90.9 kilograms

To Calculate height in meters change height to inches and multiply by 0.0254 and then square:Example:

5'8 individual     68 inches x 0.0254=1.7272 meters

                  1.7272 X 1.7272=2.9832 meters

Next: Divide your weight by kg by your hgt in meters squared: 90.9/2.9832=30 BMI

To determine your current caloric intake use the numbers below:

| Age: | Males: | Females: |
|------|--------|----------|
| 15-18 | (17.5 x weight)+651 | (12.2 x weight)+746 |
| 19-30 | (15.3 x weight)+679 | (14.7 x weight)+496 |
| 31-60 | (11.6 x weight)+879 | (8.7 x weight)+829 |
| over 60 | (13.5 x weight)+487 | (10.5 x weight)+596 |

**Example**:

21 year old standing 6'0, weighing 220 lbs. Desired Wgt.Loss: 36 lbs.

Current BMI=29.9            Desired BMI: 25

Current caloric intake=3,000      Reduced caloric intake: 1,300

Calculations: 220/2.2=100 kilograms

Height: 72 inches x 0.0254 =1.8288 meters
1.83 (meters) x 1.83 (meters)=3.34 (meters squared)

100 kilograms / 3.34 meters=29.9 BMI
100 kilograms x 16.3=1,630 calories+599=2,229 calories need to remain at 220 lbs. 100 kilograms x 30.0=3,000 actual calories you are consuming thus resulting in gain. 3,000—1,300=1,700 daily reduction in calories x 7 days weekly=11,900 decrease 11,900 caloric decrease / 3,500 (1 lb.)=3.4 pound possible weekly wgt. Loss.

## Ideal body weight:

(Desired BMI) 25 x 3.34 (hgt. in inches)= 83.50 pounds
83.50 x 2.2 kilograms=187.7 lbs. (IBW)
220 (actual weight)—183.7 (ideal body weight=36.3 lbs. Overweight
36.3 lbs. Overweight/3.4 weekly weight loss=10.6 weeks

*THESE CALCULATION ARE NOT EXACT AND INDIVIDUAL WEIGHT LOSS WILL VARY. WEIGHT LOSS IS PREDICATED ON MANY FACTORS SUCH AS PERCENT FAT INTAKE, GENETICS, BMR, ACTIVITY LEVEL AND CALORIC INTAKE.*

# *APPENDIX C*

**Contract with self for Behavior Modification Program:**

*I _____, am contracting with myself to begin and follow a nutritional/behavior modification/conscious eating/physical fitness program to work toward improving my health and reaching my weight loss goals. I list the below long-term goals as my motivation for change.*

*I.   PLEASE LIST YOUR LONG-TERM GOALS HERE:*

*1._____*

*2._____*

My program plan is as follows:

Activities for increased activity levels & decrease caloric intake:

1._____

2._____

3._____

4._____

My program will begin on _____,My program includes the below listed schedule of short-term goals and rewards.

Short-term Goals   Frequency/Duration   Reward for Completion:

_____

_____

_____

_____

_____

_____

_____

_____

_____

_____

_____          _____
      **signature**                                  **date**

# APPENDIX D

Basic Fitness Assessment Survey: (Please fill out and keep for your records) This self-assessment could give your insight into your current level of motivation.

I weigh more than I would like to.
     True_____Somewhat True_____False_____
I put off doing things most of the time.
     True_____Somewhat True_____False_____
I enjoy my free time.
     True_____Somewhat True_____False_____
I feel unattractive.
     True_____Somewhat True_____False_____
I am self-conscious about my weight.
     True_____Somewhat True_____False_____
I feel fat most of the time.
     True_____Somwwhat True_____False_____
I am self conscious about being in public.
     True_____Somewhat True_____False_____
Fats and sweets are a big problem for me.
     True_____Somewhat True_____False_____
I would like to be more healthy.
     True_____Somewhat True_____False_____
My weight causes me great dissappointment.
     True_____Somewhat True_____False_____
When I am bored or depressed I eat.

True_____Somewhat True_____False_____

I do not know what hunger feels like.

True_____Somewhat True_____False_____

I wake up feeling tired.

True_____Somewhat True_____False_____

Perception of your physical appearance.

Attractive_____ Fair_____ Unattractive _____

How do you feel most of the time?

Happy___Angry___Depressed_____Somewhat   Happy___Somewhat Depressed___

What types of food are you eating?

_____

_____

_____

_____

Are you currently using any meal replacements drinks, bars, etc.,etc.?

Yes_____ No_____ if yes, list them _____

_____

Are you currently exercising? Yes_____ No_____ Some of the time_____ if yes, what type of exercises are you performing?

_____

_____

How Often do you engage in weekly physical activities?

No. Days:_____ Lenth of time spent daily:_____.

*AFTER COMPLETION OF THIS SELF SURVEY YOU SHOULD HAVE A CLEAR PICTURE OF YOUR ATTITUDE, MOTIVATION AND CURRENT OUTLOOK AS IT RELATES TO FITNESS LEVEL.*

# *APPENDIX E*

Creating Your Behavioral Modification Program:

Name:_____Starting Date: _____
Current Weight: _____(kg) Height: _____(meters)
BMI:_____ Pants/Skirt/Dress size:_____Current Shirt/Blouse
size: _____ Waist:_____ Current Resting Metabolic
Rate:_____ this is your current daily intake. Weight (pounds)
_____/2.2=_____(kilograms) X 30=_____actual calories Actual
calories eaten daily _____ X 7 days weekly=_____. Insert
weekly calories _____/3,500 (1 lb.)=_____ possible weekly
lost. Current weight: _____(pounds)—_____(pounds) Your
desired/goal weight=_____(lbs.overweight)/_____(weekly
lost)=_____weeks to goal wgt.

I. Reason(s) For Desired Weight Loss:

_____
_____
_____
_____
_____

II. List and Describe Your Previous Attempts and Experience with
Weight Loss.

_____
_____
_____
_____

_____

_____

_____

_____

_____

_____

## III. Goal Setting: An Essential First Step:

Goal setting is an important aspect and strategy for encouragement when attempting to lose weight. It helps you to become more focused & self-directed. Through goalassessment you can identify, set and reach your goals by breaking them down complex into a series of small successive behaviroal steps. Because you are deciding the goals the commitment should be reached.

**Goal Identification:** The initial step is to identify the goals that you want to reach. Goals are set and you begin to take action to reach the desired goals. Goals are different from results, you may not have the immediate or exact results you desire, but you should remain focused and continue on the path to reaching the goals set. List your goals and define your goal behavior. Ex:I will eat more fruits & vegetables daily. or, I will become more active.

1._____

_____

2._____

_____

3._____

_____

4._____

_____

**Goal Importance:** The 2<sup>nd</sup> step in goal assessment is the importance and meaning of the goal, in essence who is the goal important to. If you are pursuing weight loss for someone other than yourself or for other external reasons; it is unlikely that it will be successful long-term. Unimportnat goals are rarely, if ever, reached. Negative/External reasoning: I will lose weight for my spouse or boyfriend/girlfriend. Positive/Internal reasoning: I will begin incresing my activity levels and healthy conscious eating, so that I may attain and maintain a healthy weight thus improving my overall health.

**Plan to Measure Short-Term Goal Progression:** Remember any new undertaking requires an initial "fit-in", time requirement phase. This time is needed to incorporate your new activities into your normal daily lifestyle, whereas it becomes automatic or second-nature. So give yourself ample time to incorporate strategies into your life that allow you to reach your goals.

Below list your strategic plan for change:

_____

_____

_____

_____

_____

IV. Activities that you plan to incorporate into your daily lifestyle to increase your activity level:

| Activity | Frequency | Duration | Intensity |
|----------|-----------|----------|-----------|
| 1. | | | |
| 2. | | | |
| 3. | | | |
| 4. | | | |
| 5. | | | |

Reward(s) for reaching short-term goals:

_____

_____

_____

_____

_____

### List long-term goals:

1. _____

2. _____

3. _____

4. _____

5. _____

Reward for reaching long-term goals:

_____

_____

_____

_____

V. I will replace old habits with new habits beginning:_____

**Old Habits:        New Habits:  Desired          Results:__**

1. _____

2. _____

3. _____

VI. Do You Eat Breakfast Daily? Yes_____ No_____ Sometimes_____

if your answer is no, why not? _____

_____

How many times a day are you eating? Less than 2 _____
2X-3X _____ 4X-6X _____ more than 6X _____

What time is your first meal? _____ 2nd meal _____
3rd_____4th _____ 5th meal _____ 6th _____

List the types of foods that you are eating for breakfast:

_____
_____
_____
_____

List the types of foods that you are eating for morning snacks:

_____
_____
_____
_____

List the types of foods that you are eating for lunch:

_____
_____
_____
_____

List the types of foods that you are eating for late evening snacks:

_____
_____
_____
_____

List the types of foods that you are eating for dinner/supper:

_____
_____
_____
_____

Are you a late night snacker? Yes: _____ No:_____ Not Sure:_____ If yes, list the foods that you are eating as late night snacks:

_____

_____

_____

_____

List below the foods/snacks that you feel you can definitely take out of your daily food consumption and replace with healthier selections:

_____

_____

_____

_____

Previous Food Selection:    Replacement Food Choice:    Reward:

1. _____

2._____

3. _____

4. _____

5. _____

6. _____

7. _____

8. _____

9. _____

10._____

Perceived Obstacles/Roadblocks That You Feel Will Slow Down Your Progress: These obstacles/roadblocks are not insurmountable, although they often seem so. Realize change can occur when some of these obstacles/roadblocks, (whether real or perceived) are kept under control. Learn additional skills, acquire new information to assist you with handling problematic and/or uncomfortable situations. Below list the obstacles that you feel will hamper your weight loss efforts.

---

---

---

---

---

**List Your Plan to Combat/Overcome these Obstacles/Roadblocks.**

---

---

---

---

---

# *Glossary*

**Acid Reflux**—When stomach acid backs up into your food pipe causing a burning sensation to the back of your throat and chest.

**Adipocyte**—Fat cell.

**Adipose Tissue**—Tissue in the human body where fat is stored.

**Amino Acids**—Component of protein used to build muscle.

**Bariatric**—Branch of medicine specializing in obesity.

**Basal Metabolic Rate(BMR)**—Utilization of energy for vital(daytime) cellular activity. **Calorie**-The amount of heat necessary to raise the temperature of water one degree celsius.

**Carbohydrate**—Principal energy for body; includes sugars; starches; pastas; breads.

**Cardiorespiratory System**—The body components that consist of your respiratory system, including your lungs and heart that deliver oxygen to your muscles, cells,and peripheral.

**Diet**—Balanced eating from a variety of foods.

**Disaccharides**—Simple sugar; two sugar molecule.

**Dumping Syndrome**—The small bowel is irritated causing the bowel to cramp; producing diarrhea, abdominal pain with nausea and headache, flushing, and palpitations, and an overall feeling of malaise.

**Enzymes**—Are proteins responsible for digestion.

**Essential Amino Acids**—Provides all the necessary proteins your body needs.

**Fat cell**—A cell containing adipose tissue.

**Glucose**—A simple sugar that is used by your body as it's basic fuel/energy.

**Glycogen**—Complex carbohydrates that are stored in your muscles and liver and is used for energy.

**Healthy Conscious Eating**—The quantity of food, the quality of food and the times that you eat those foods.

**Heart Burn**—See Acid Reflux.

**High-density Lipoprotein**— Fats that carry cholesterol away from your arteries.

**Hunger Backlash**—When you starve yourself and become extremely hungry later, thus overeating.

**Hypercellular Obesity**—Instance where one's fat cell increase in number.

**Hyperglycemia**—Increased glucose level in your blood.

**Hypertension**—Chronic abnormality high blood pressure; greater than 140/90.

**Hypertrophic Obesity**—Instance where one's fat cells increase in size.

**Hypothalamus**—A part of your brain that controls bodily functions including appetite.

**Isometric Activities**—Activities using stable objects; force without movement.

**Isotonic Activities**—Activities that utilizes force resulting in movement.

**Ketone Body**—Accumulates in your body when fat is used as energy instead of glucose.

**Lactic Acid**—A metabolic acid that comes from the breakdown of glucose & glycogen usage during high and low intensity levels of activities.

**Laparoscopic Surgery**—Video surgery using multiple small incisions.

**Lean Body Mass**—The nonfat components of your body (skeletal & vital organs).

**Lipids**—A fat like substance such as triglycerides.

**Lipoprotein**—A substance within your body that transport fat.

**Low-Density-Lipoproteins (LDL)**—Fats that transport cholesterol to your body's organs and tissue that utilizes it.

**Metabolic Rate**—Metabolism per unit time esp., as estimated by food consumption, energy released as heat or oxygen used in metabolic processes; (Merriam-Webster's Medical Dictionary 1995 edition).

**Metabolism**—Your body's ability to utilize food and nutrients for energy.

**Monosaccharides**—Simple sugar; one molecule.

**Nutrition**—The total process of eating and digestion of food, vitamins and minerals for health.

**Obesity**—Excessive body fat.

**Osmotic Concentration**—The concentration or number of food particles per ounce of the food mixture.

**Overweight**—A body weight above recommendation using BMI.

**Plaque**—A fatty substance that builds up and can deposit on your arterial walls.

**Polysaccharide**—Many sugar molecule.

**Polyunsaturated Fats**—Constituents of margarine and olive oils.

**Progressive Overload**—A method of stressing your body physically to induce positive physiological changes.

**Protein**—Basic anatomical and physiological building blocks; important for growth of hair and nails & degenerative bones and tissue repair.

**Resting Metabolic Rate (RMR)**—The cellular energy needed to sustain bodily functions.

**Satiety**—The feeling and satisfaction of fullness.

**Saturated Fats**-Animal fats believed to increase cholesterol levels.

**Self Talk**—The internal conversation that one has with one's self.

**Stress**—The physiological, emotional and behavioral response to a
  situation.

**Stressor**—A situation(s) or event that produces stress.

**Sugar**—Occurs naturally in food; instant energy; no nutritional properties.

**Target Heart Rate**—A level of calculated exertion to enhance fitness.

**Unsaturated Fats**—Animal fats; meats, eggs,et.,